D1425326

WB18 NIC

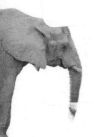

# Mnemonics
## for MRCP

Timothy Nicholson

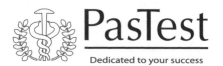

PasTest

Dedicated to your success

© 2006 PASTEST LTD
Egerton Court
Parkgate Estate
Knutsford
Cheshire
WA16 8DX

Telephone: 01565 752000

All rights reserved. No part of this publication may be reproduced, stored in a retrieval system, or transmitted, in any form or by any means, electronic, mechanical, photocopying, recording or otherwise without the prior permission of the copyright owner.

First Published 2006

ISBN: 1 904627 98 6
ISBN: 978 1904 627 982

A catalogue record for this book is available from the British Library.

The information contained within this book was obtained by the author from reliable sources. However, while every effort has been made to ensure its accuracy, no responsibility for loss, damage or injury occasioned to any person acting or refraining from action as a result of information contained herein can be accepted by the publishers or author.

---

### PasTest Revision Books and Intensive Courses

PasTest has been established in the field of postgraduate medical education since 1972, providing revision books and intensive study courses for doctors preparing for their professional examinations.

Books and courses are available for the following specialties:

**MRCGP, MRCP Parts 1 and 2, MRCPCH Parts 1 and 2, MRCPsych, MRCS, MRCOG Parts 1 and 2, DRCOG, DCH, FRCA, PLAB Parts 1 and 2.**

For further details contact:

PasTest, Freepost, Knutsford, Cheshire WA16 7BR

**Tel: 01565 752000**   **Fax: 01565 650264**
**www.pastest.co.uk**   **enquiries@pastest.co.uk**

---

Text typeset and designed by Type Study, Scarborough, North Yorkshire

Printed and bound in the UK by MPG Books Ltd., Bodmin, Cornwall

# Mnemonic

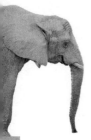

1753, from the Greek *mnemonikos* 'of or pertaining to memory,' from *mnemon* (gen. *mnemonos*) 'remembering, mindful,' from *mnasthai* 'remember.'

*Mnemosyne,* lit. 'memory, remembrance,' was a Titaness, mother of the Muses.

# Contents

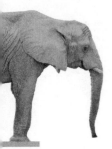

# Acknowledgements

For Helen and her patience.

Thank you to the following for their help and advice:

Paul Dilworth
Fahad Farooqi
Jack Galliford
Thomas Galliford
Andrew Jaques

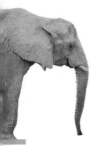

# Preface

I have collected and made up these mnemonics over many years and found them very useful in preparing for the MRCP, as did my colleagues who I shared them with.

Learning long 'dry' lists is difficult, especially when you're having to squeeze studying into bus/train/tube journeys or the odd moment free in the evening after work. The process of making mnemonics is in itself a good way of learning, as you are continually thinking about the topic in hand. Your own mnemonics are often the best as they are specific, and therefore more memorable, to you. Therefore, use this book as a springboard by adapting these mnemonics or making your own ones up.

Good mnemonics are obviously relevant to the condition/list, striking or memorable in other ways. The hardest thing to do is to get the lists in order of the most common or relevant answers, especially for mnemonics to be used in clinical exams such as as PACES. It will look odd reciting rare causes first, and do you no favours if you forget the end of the mnemonic or are interrupted by your examiner before you finish the list! On this note, leave learning the detailed mnemonics until you have covered the basics.

Good luck with the exam!

**Timothy Nicholson**

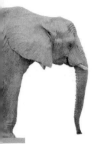

# Introduction

## Key

After the title of each mnemonic, there is a key to help identify which mnemonics will be useful for which parts of the exam.

A symbol is given for each part of the exam that the mnemonic is relevant to. 1, 2 or 3 stripes through this then denote the level of relevance. For example:

Part 1 **Part 1** This denotes that the mnemonic is useful for the Part 1 – the symbol denotes that the information in this mnemonic is *very commonly* tested and therefore *particularly* worth spending time learning.

Part 2 **Part 2** This denotes that the mnemonic is useful for the Part 2 written paper – the symbol denotes that it is commonly tested and worth spending time learning.

PACES **PACES** This denotes that the mnemonic is useful for the PACES exam – the symbol denotes that it is less commonly tested and only worth spending time remembering after the more commonly tested information/mnemonics have been learnt.

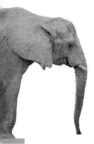

# Abbreviations

| | | | |
|---|---|---|---|
| ABPA | Allergic broncho-pulmonary aspergillosis | CJD | Creutzfeldt–Jakob disease |
| ACE | Angiotensin converting enzyme | CLL | Chronic lymphoblastic leukaemia |
| ACTH | Adrenocorticotrophin | CML | Chronic myeloid leukaemia |
| ADH | Antidiuretic hormone | CMV | Cytomegalovirus |
| ADHD | Attention deficit hyperactivity disorder | COPD | Chronic obstructive pulmonary disease |
| AF | Atrial fibrillation | CRF | Chronic renal failure |
| AIDP | Acute inflammatory demyelinating polyneuropathy | CRP | C-reactive protein |
| | | CSF | Cerebrospinal fluid |
| | | CVA | Cerebrovascular accident |
| | | CXR | Chest X-ray |
| AIDS | Acquired immunodeficiency syndrome | DIC | Disseminated intravascular coagulation |
| ALT | Alanine aminotransferase | DKA | Diabetic ketoacidosis |
| AML | Acute myeloid leukaemia | DVT | Deep venous thrombosis |
| ANCA | Antineutrophil cytoplasmic antibody | Dx | Diagnosis |
| | | EAA | Extrinsic allergic alveolitis |
| APC | Activated protein C | EBV | Epstein–Barr virus |
| APTT | Activated partial thromboplastin time | ECG | Electrocardiogram |
| | | ESR | Erythrocyte sedimentation rate |
| ARF | Acute renal failure | | |
| ASD | Atrial septal defect | FISH | Fluorescent in situ hybridisation |
| ASOT | Antistreptolysin O titre | | |
| AST | Aspartate transaminase | FSH | Follicle-stimulating hormone |
| ATN | Acute tubular necrosis | G6PD | Glucose 6-phosphate dehydrogenase |
| AVM | Arteriovenous malformation | | |
| BMR | Basic metabolic rate | GnRH | Gonadotrophin-releasing hormone |
| CABG | Coronary artery bypass graft | | |
| CAH | Congenital adrenal hyperplasia | Hb | Haemoglobin |
| | | HF | Heart failure |
| CCF | Congestive cardiac failure | HHT | Hereditary haemorrhagic telangiectasia |
| CFA | Cryptogenic fibrosing alveolitis | | |
| | | HMG | 3-Hydroxy-3-methylglutaryl coenzyme A |
| CIDP | Chronic inflammatory demyelinating polyneuropathy | | |
| | | HOCM | Hypertrophic obstructive cardiomyopathy |

| | | | |
|---|---|---|---|
| HR | Heart rate | PDA | Patent ductus arteriosus |
| HRT | Hormone replacement therapy | PE | Pulmonary embolism |
| | | PMA | Peroneal muscular atrophy |
| HSMN | Hereditary sensory motor neuropathy | PNH | Paroxysmal nocturnal haemoglobinuria |
| 5-HT | 5-Hydroxytryptamine | PRV | Polycythaemia rubra vera |
| HTN | Hypertension | PT | Prothrombin time |
| Hx | History | PTH | Parathyroid hormone |
| HZV | Herpes zoster virus | PVD | Peripheral vascular disease |
| IBD | Inflammatory bowel disease | RBC | Red blood cell |
| IGF | Insulin-like growth factor | REM | Rapid eye movement |
| IHD | Ischaemic heart disease | RTA | Renal tubular acidosis |
| IMN | Infectious mononucleosis | RV | Right ventricle |
| INO | Internuclear ophthalmoplegia | RVH | Right ventricular hypertrophy |
| ITP | Idiopathic thrombocytopenic purpura | Rx | Treatment/therapy |
| | | SAH | Subarachnoid haemorrhage |
| ITU | Intensive therapy unit | SBE | Subacute bacterial endocarditis |
| IUGR | Intrauterine growth retardation | SCA | Spinocerebellar ataxia |
| LA | Left atrium | SLE | Systemic lupus erythematosus |
| LBBB | Left bundle branch block | | |
| LDH | Lactate dehydrogenase | SSRI | Selective serotonin-reuptake inhibitors |
| LFT | Liver function test | | |
| LH | Luteinising hormone | SVC | Superior vena cava |
| LMN | Lower motor neurone | $T_3$ | Tri-iodothyronine |
| LVH | Left ventricular hypertrophy | $T_4$ | Thyroxine |
| MAOI | Monoamine oxidase inhibitors | TB | Tuberculosis |
| MEN | Multiple endocrine neoplasia | TCA | Tricyclic antidepressant |
| MI | Myocardial infarction | TIA | Transient ischaemic attack |
| MLF | Medial longitudinal fasciculus | TNF | Tumour necrosis factor |
| MS | Multiple sclerosis | TTP | Thrombotic thrombocytopaenic purpura |
| NMDA | *N*-Methyl-D-asparate | | |
| NSAIDs | Non-steroidal anti-inflammatory drugs | UC | Ulcerative colitis |
| | | UMN | Upper motor neurone |
| OCD | Obsessive compulsive disorder | UTI | Urinary tract infection |
| | | VDRL | Venereal disease research laboratory |
| OCP | Oral contraceptive pill | | |
| PAN | Polyarteritis nodosa | VIP | Vasoactive intestinal polypeptide |
| PBC | Primary biliary cirrhosis | | |
| PCOS | Polycystic ovary disease | VSD | Ventricular septal defect |
| PCP | Pneumocystis carinii pneumonia | WCC | White cell count |
| | | WPW | Wolf–Parkinson–White |
| PCV | Packed cell volume | | |

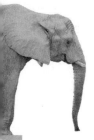

# 1. Syndromes

Angelman syndrome

**ANGEL WOMAN**

| | |
|---|---|
| **A** | **A**rms of a puppet[1] |
| **N** | **N**ever sleep |
| **G** | **G**ait ataxia |
| **E** | **E**pilepsy: characteristic **EEG** |
| **L** | **L**ow IQ: severe[2] mental retardation |
| | |
| **W** | **W**ide-spaced teeth |
| **O** | **O**rofacial abnormalities[3] |
| **M** | **M**icrocephaly |
| **A** | **A**miable/**A**lways laughing[4] |
| **N** | **N**o (or little) speech |

**notes**

The mnemonic is changed from Angel 'man' to 'woman' to remind you that the majority of these patients have deletions in their maternal chromosome 16q. Paternal (uniparental) disomy accounts for a smaller number of cases. Prader–Willi (see p. 6) is the opposite, being caused by deletion of maternal chromosome 15q or paternal uniparental disomy

1 Arm posture is characteristic: elbows and wrists in flexion; creates look of a puppet*

2 Lower IQ than those with Prader–Willli, who have moderate mental retardation

3 Large mouth, magroglossia, wide-spaced teeth; also maxillary hypoplasia (creates prognathism; protruding mandible)

4 Laughter is mostly inappropriate*

*These two features lead to the phrase 'happy puppet', which is used to describe people with this syndrome; they also clap hands a lot like a puppet

**Part 1** Di George's syndrome

## CATCH 22 situations are stressful and can lead to mental health problems!

### CATCH 22

C   Cardiac abnormalities[1]
A   Abnormal (dysmorphic) face[2]
T   Thymic hypoplasia ($\Rightarrow \downarrow$ T cells[3]; especially CD4)
C   Cleft palate
H   Hypocalcaemia[4]
22  Chromosome **22**[5]

### Predisposes to mental health problems[6]

**notes**

aka 'Velo-Cardio-Facial Syndrome'. Genetic cause of defective branchial arch (3rd and 4th pharyngeal pouches) development which then causes defective thymic development and the other abnormalities. The complete syndrome is listed above but partial forms exist

1   Congenital malformations; especially interrupted aortic arch and truncus arteriosus
2   Characteristic facies are small, low-set ears, elongated face, almond-shaped eyes and wide nose
3   $\downarrow$ T cells causes $\uparrow$ infections (especially mucocutaneous candidiasis, PCP, mycobacteria) and chronic diarrhoea; bone marrow transplant can overcome this problem
4   Hypocalcaemia occurs due to $\downarrow$ PTH – these patients fail to develop parathyroid glands; often severe and leads to patients presenting with convulsions in neonatal period
5   The defect on chromosome 22; this is a microdeletion on 22q11 which can be detected by the FISH technique
6   Psychiatric consequences are common, ranging from learning difficulties, to OCD symptoms, to presentations similar to schizophrenia or bipolar disorder

## Edward's syndrome

### EDWARD'S SCISSORHANDS

**E**  **E**ighteenth chromosome (trisomy): cause of syndrome!
**D**  **D**orsiflexion of hallux occurs in all toes
**W**  **W**edge-shaped base of skull: prominent occiput
**A**  **A**ortic and other cardiac abnormalities[1]
**R**  **R**ockerbottom feet[2]/**R**enal abnormalities are common[3]
**D**  **D**iaphragmatic hernias/**D**ermatoglyphic abnormalities[4]
**S**  **S**mall nails and sternum

**Scissor hands**: index and little fingers overlap the middle two
*'Edward scissor hands' is a rather strange (yet critically
acclaimed!) film with Johnny Depp, who plays a misunderstood
man with scissors for hands!*

> Other features are low set ears and micrognathia. Aplasia of radius, facial
> clefts and exomphalos can each occur in 20% of cases. Dislocation of hips is
> common
>
> Patients are born of low birth weight (IUGR) and with hypotonia. Half die
> before 2 months (99% before 10 years). Profound mental retardation
> manifests itself if the patient lives long enough
>
> 1  Increased incidence of VSD and PDA
> 2  'Rockerbottom feet': vertical talus causes convex foot with prominent heel
> 3  Renal abnormalities: horseshoe kidney and hydronephrosis
> 4  Increased number of arch patterns

## Fetal alcohol syndrome

### FACIAL

**F**  **F**acies[1]
**A**  **A**DHD[2]
**C**  **C**ardiac abnormalities[3]
**I**  **I**ntestinal abnormalities (especially hernias)
**A**  **A**uditory abnormalities
**L**  **L**ow IQ and birth weight

> **notes**
>
> 1 Microcephaly, midface hypoplasia, flattened philtrum, thin upper lip, cleft palate, jaw abnormalities (retrognathia in infancy then micrognathia or relative prognathism in adolescence), low nasal bridge, small widely spaced eyes, strabismus, ptosis, short palpebral fissures, posterior rotation of the ears
> 2 ADHD is attention deficit hyperactivity disorder; also many other cognitive and behavioural problems
> 3 Most common congenital problems: ASD/VSD, Fallot's tetralogy, PDA, great vessel abnormalities and dextrocardia
>
> NB Alcohol in pregnancy causes widespread damage and affects most tissues; urogenital, renal, musculoskeletal and ocular abnormalities also common

**Part 1** Homocystinuria versus Marfan's (differences)

Homocystinuria has the following features (that Marfan's doesn't):

**High:**   **T**hromboembolism (DVT/PE)
       **H**eart complications[1]
       **E**pilepsy

**Low:**   **B**one density (ie osteoporosis)
       **L**ens[2]
       **I**Q
       **N**umbers in pedigrees[3]
       **D**etached retina[4]

***BLIND** reminds you of the eye complications and the fact that BLIND is underneath the word THE reminds you it is the cause of things being lowered!*

> **notes**
>
> Otherwise these two syndromes look similar, with the same body habitus and skeletal features
>
> 1 IHD, aortic regurgitation (and dissection) or mitral prolapse
> 2 Dislocation is down (and in): in Marfan's it is up (and out)
> 3 Autosomal recessive inheritance; Marfan's = autosomal dominant
> 4 Detached retina is the only one in this list that doesn't fit with the list that it is in – it is of increased frequency in homocystinuria!

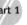

## art 1 Hurler's (and Hunter's*) syndrome

### THICK BONES

| | |
|---|---|
| **T** | **T**hrills (heart murmurs)[1] |
| **H** | **H**epatosplenomegaly |
| **I** | **I**ncreased head:body ratio[2] |
| **C** | **C**orneal **C**louding[3] + papilloedema |
| **K** | **K**yphosis |

**Bones** ↑diameter of bones ('Stocky'!)

*Thick bones are a feature of the illness and thick also refers (in a politically incorrect way) to the low IQ seen in this syndrome; developmental delay also seen in children before IQ is measured*

1 Thickened valves (also heart failure, myocardial rigidity and narrowing of arteries)
2 Large head with frontal bossing
3 Differentiates this condition from Hunter's syndrome*

Hurler's syndrome is a genetic (autosomal recessive) disorder of mucopolysaccharide metabolism (lysosomal storage)

Other features: protruberant abdomen, umbilical hernias, short stature ('dwarfism') and generally 'coarse' facial features (hence old name 'Gargoylism')

*Hunter's syndrome: X-linked recessive mucopolysaccharidosis with almost identical features apart from:

- No corneal clouding
- Have nodes over the scapulae

## art 1 Kallman's syndrome

### GONAD

| | |
|---|---|
| **G** | **G**nRH deficiency[1] |
| **O** | **O**lfactory impairment: anosmia (or severe hyposmia) |
| **N** | **N**o colour vision |
| **A** | **A**bnormal face[2] |
| **D** | **D**eafness (sensorineural) |

> Genetic syndrome: can be X or autosomal recessive. Two-thirds have no family history and are spontaneous mutations
>
> *Should be suspected in anyone with delayed puberty and ↓ sense of smell of normal stature*
>
> 1 Isolated **Gonad**otrophin-releasing hormone deficiency: caused by failure of migration of GnRH neurones from site of origin in the nose ⇒ ↓ **Gonad**otrophins (LH, FSH and sex steroids) ⇒ delayed puberty and ↓ fertility *but normal (or even ↑)* stature
> 2 Midline face abnormalities: cleft palate/lip and high arched palate
>
> Other: cardiac defects (most congenital ones)

---

**Part 1** Phenylketonuria

---

### Dumb blonde

**Dumb:**  Mental retardation
**Blonde:** Blonde hair
Blue eyes
Pale skin (hypopigmentation)

> Other features: **irritable** (mood) + **itchy** (eczema)
>
> Genetics: mutations of phenylalanine hydroxylase gene on chromosome 12, which normally converts phenylalanine into tyrosine, causing excess phenylalanine. Diagnosis is by Guthrie (heel prick) test

---

**Part 1** Prader–Willi syndrome

---

### PRADER WILLY

| | |
|---|---|
| **P** | **P**alpebral fissure abnormality ('almond shape') |
| **R** | **R**ound face/obese |
| **A** | **A**ngry outbursts[1] |
| **D** | **D**ownturned mouth |
| **E** | **E**at excessively[2] |
| **R** | **R**educed tone |
| **Willy** | small genitals/cryptorchidism[3] |

notes

Willy also makes you remember the deletion is of the paternal chromosome (15q). Maternal (uniparental) disomy accounts for a smaller number of cases. Angelman (see p. 1) is the opposite, being caused by deletion of maternal chromosome 15q or paternal uniparental disomy

1 Stubborness/rages; also learning difficulties (moderate to severe) and verbal perseverance (sticks to favourite topics!)
2 Overwhelming compulsion to eat (hyperphagia)
3 Also small hands/feet and small in general (ie height!)

# Turner's syndrome*

## SHORT AND WIDE

**S** **S**eptal defects (VSD, ASD)
**H** **H**ypertension[1]/**Hi**p fractures (↑ risk of)
**O** **O**steoporosis
**R** **R**enal anomalies[2]
**T** **T**hyroid abnormalities[3]

**A** **A**orta and **A**ortic valve abnormalities[4]
**N** **N**ail hypoplasia/**N**aevi excess on skin
**D** **D**iabetes (↑ risk of type II)

**W** **W**eb-shaped neck[5]
**I** **I**nflammatory bowel disease (↑ risk of Crohn's/UC)
**D** **D**ysgenesis of ovaries: 'streak ovaries'[6]
**E** **E**ar[7]/**E**ye[8] abnormalities

*Affected individuals are* **short** *and* **wide**

**Short** *refers to:*

- *Stature: results from slow growth as child, then absent pubertal growth spurt. Scoliosis is also common and can contribute*
- *4th metatarsals and metacarpals: can suggest the diagnosis if seen*

**Wide** *refers to:*

- *Wide body, ie overweight/obese*
- *Widely space nipples: due to broad (= 'shield') chest*
- *Wide carrying angle = 'Cubitus valgus'*

notes

1 Hypertension: can be primary or secondary to coarctation, renal abnormalities or obesity/diabetes

2 Renal abnormalities: congenital anomalies, eg 'Horseshoe' kidneys; also ↑ incidence of UTIs

3 Thyroid abnormalities: up to 50% anti-thyroid antibody positive; 10–30% develop hypothyroidism (often associated with goitre)

4 Aortic coarctaction (±dissection) and aortic stenosis (or bicuspid valve)

5 Webbed neck: due to fetal lymphoedema** which also causes the characteristic low posterior hairline. Webbed neck also seen in Noonan's syndrome (along with low IQ, HOCM and pulmonary stenosis)

6 Ovarian dysgenesis causes primary hypogonadism and amenorrhoea; secondary sexual characteristics are poorly developed

7 Ears: are low set. Hearing loss (due to otosclerosis) and otitis media are common

8 Eyes: ptosis, amblyopia, strabismus and cataracts common; can also have epicanthal folds

*This mnemonic is very inclusive and a bit cumbersome for the PACES exam and consequently not a good one to try and remember unless already learnt for Part 1. Just remember the key points of 'Short' and 'Wide' and to look for the syndromic appearance (nipples, neck, naevi, 4th metatarsals/metacarpals) if the patient is short stature. You can make a particularly clever diagnosis if you see this syndrome in someone who has a goitre, aortic stenosis, coarctation or ASD/VSD

**Lymphoedema: occurs at any age and is suggestive of the syndrome on fetal ultrasonography; especially in hands and feet which together with the nail changes cause 'sausage-shaped' fingers and toes; when this resolves it can lead to loose skin folds (especially in the neck) known as 'cutis laxa'

### Genetics

Turner's syndrome patients are females of genotype 45XO; this results from non-disjunction of the X chromosomes from either parent. Most 'pure' forms are spontaneously aborted but of those that aren't most are 'mosaics', which means some of their cells are normal, ie 46XX, or more rarely 45XY. In normal 46XX females one copy of the X chromosome in each cell is functionally inactivated (by lyonisation) causing a Barr body, the absence of which is diagnostic of Turner's

NB IQ is normal and this is an often asked question that catches people out!

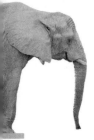

# 2. Cardiology

## Pericarditis

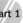

### CARDIAC RUB

| | |
|---|---|
| **C** | **C**oxsackie virus[1]/**C**oronary syndromes |
| **A** | **A**utoimmune[2] |
| **R** | **R**heumatic fever |
| **D** | **D**rugs[3] |
| **I** | **I**nvasive techniques[4] |
| **A** | **A**ortic aneurysm |
| **C** | **C**ancer: metastases in pericardium |
| **R** | **R**adiotherapy |
| **U** | **U**raemia (ie renal failure!) |
| **B** | **B**lunt injury/trauma[5] |

---

**notes**

1 And other infections: especially other viruses, TB and parasites
2 Autoimmune causes:
   - Post MI; Dressler's syndrome
   - Connective tissue diseases: especially SLE, scleroderma, mixed connective tissue diseases
   - Hypothyroidism
3 Hydralazine (causes 'lupus-like' syndrome), anticoagulants, procainamide
4 For example, post cardiac catheterisation (angiograms, angioplasty, pacemaker insertions) or surgery
5 Blunt trauma most common; especially seat belt injuries

---

# Rheumatic fever

**Revised (Duckett) Jones Criteria:**

**ARTHRITIS Can Skip EveryWhere; Legs Around Patella Are Frequently Preferred**

| MAJOR | **Arthritis** | **A**rthritis |
|---|---|---|
| | **Can** | **C**arditis[1] |
| | **Skip** | **S**ubcutaneous nodules (= 'Aschoff' nodules) |
| | **Every** | **E**rythema marginatum[2] |
| | **Where** | **W**rithing[3] = Chorea |
| MINOR | **Legs** | **L**eukocytosis |
| | **Around** | **A**rthr-**A**lgia[4] |
| | **Patellae**[5] | **P**R interval prolongation |
| | **Are** | **A**cute phase response[6] |
| | **Frequently** | **F**ever |
| | **Preferred** | **P**revious rheumatic fever |

*Arthritis in rheumatic fever is described as 'fleeting': as the inflammation of one joint recedes another joint become involved, therefore the arthritis 'skips everywhere'! Leg joints (especially knees[3] and ankles) are the most commonly affected*

---

**notes**

**Diagnosis**

- Requires evidence of antecedent streptococcal infection such as Hx of recent scarlet fever, positive antistreptolysin O titre (ASOT) or throat culture for group A *Streptococcus*, **plus** 2 major criteria or 1 major + 2 minor criteria

1 Carditis in this context is defined as:
  - New or changed murmur
  - Development of CCF or cardiac enlargement
  - Development of pericardial effusion and ECG changes of pericarditis (saddle-shaped ST elevation) or myocarditis (flattened or inverted T waves), any heart block or other cardiac arrhythmias
  - Transient diastolic mitral (Carey–Coombs) murmur due to mitral valvulitis
2 Non-itchy pink rings that come and go (for up to several months) on the trunk and inner limbs

3  'Writhes' is also a mnemonic for chorea (see p. 70). In the context of rheumatic fever, chorea is sometimes called 'Syndenham's chorea' or 'St. Vitus' dance': patients are fidgety with spasmodic unintentional movements and speech is often affected

4  Not arthr-*itis*; minor swelling compared to pain!

5  Patellae = Knees!

6  ↑CRP or ESR (each is a criterion on its own)

## Fallot's tetralogy

### PROVERB

**P\***  **P**ulmonary stenosis
**R\***  **R**ight ventricular hypertrophy
**O\***  **O**verriding aorta
**V\***  **V**SD (⇒ harsh systolic murmur at left sternal edge)
**E**  **E**xercise-induced syncope is main symptom
**R**  **R**ight-sided aortic arch (in 20%)/**R**epair[1]
**B**  **B**lalock–Taussig shunt[2]

1  Total repair is the definitive surgical treatment after a Blalock–Taussig shunt

2  Blalock–Taussig 'shunt' is of (left) subclavian artery to pulmonary artery – palliative procedure often needed before total repair in order to allow increased growth of pulmonary vasculature. In older patients (the initial operations) this was the final operation as total repairs were not then possible

\*These 4 features make up the tetralogy

NB In Fallot's, quieter murmurs (of PS or VSD) often indicate worse cardiac function!

**Part 1** Long QT interval

**Part 2** **Low Electrolytes MAKES TORSADES**

**Low** ↓ Temperature or $T_4$

**Electrolytes** ↓ $Mg^{2+}/Ca^{2+}/K^+$

| | |
|---|---|
| **M** | **M**itral valve prolapse |
| **A** | **A**cute coronary syndromes or carditis |
| **K** | **K**etoconazole |
| **E** | **E**rythromycin/clarithromycin[1] |
| **S** | **S**chizophrenia Rx[2] |
| | |
| **T** | **T**erfenadine[3]/**T**amoxifen |
| **O** | **O**ne a+c antiarrhythmics[4] |
| **R** | **R**heumatic fever |
| **S** | **S**otalol, ie class III antiarrhythmics |
| **A** | **A**miodarone, ie class III antiarrhythmics |
| **D** | **D**epression Rx[5] |
| **S** | **S**ubarachnoid haemorrhage/**S**yndromes[6]/**S**leep[7] |

**notes**

↑QT interval is a risk factor for syncope, Torsades de pointes (polymorphic VT) and other ventricular arrhythmias, as well as sudden death

1 Other antibiotics are less common causes: ampicillin, septrin and pentamidine
2 All antipsychotics, to varying degrees, can ↑ QT (= neuroleptics = dopamine antagonists)
3 And to a lesser degree other non-sedating antihistamines
4 Class 1a: eg quinidine, procainamide, disopyramide
   Class 1c: eg flecainide, propafenone
   NB Class 1b (eg lidocaine) drugs do not alter QTc!
5 Especially tricyclic antidepressants (eg amitriptyline or nortriptyline)
6 Genetic syndromes:
   ● Romano–Ward: relatively common (compared to Jarvell–Lange–Nielsen), therefore can be remembered as *dominantly* inherited (chromosome 11)
   ● Jervell–Lange–Nielsen: rarer (therefore remember as recessive) and associated with congenital deafness. NB Heterozygotes are also at increased risk of arrhythmias
7 Sleep is a rare physiological cause: as are exercise, shock, stress and extremes of age

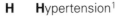

# Causes of atrial fibrillation

## HELPS TIM'S ACHES

| | |
|---|---|
| **H** | **H**ypertension[1] |
| **E** | **E**tOH – acute intoxication or chronic abuse[2] |
| **L** | **L**one (ie idiopathic) |
| **P** | **P**neumonia (+ sepsis per se)[3] |
| | |
| **T** | **T**hyrotoxicosis |
| **I** | **I**schaemic heart disease |
| **M** | **M**itral valve (stenosis > regurgitation) |
| **S** | **S**ick sinus syndrome |
| | |
| **A** | **A**berrant pathway conduction[4]/**A**SD/**A**trial myxoma |
| **C** | **C**arditis[5]/**C**ardiomyopathy/**C**ABG/**C**affeine excess |
| **H** | **H**aemochromatosis |
| **E** | **E**mbolism (ie PE) |
| **S** | **S**arcoid |

*This mnemonic does list the causes relatively well according to frequency; 'ACHES' denotes rarer causes and therefore not so important to remember and don't mention 1st in PACES exam!*

> **notes**
> 1 And other causes of LVH or dilated LA (>4.5 cm)
> 2 Chronic alcohol abuse usually causes AF via cardiomyopathy
> 3 Pulmonary malignancy is also a rare cause
> 4 Eg WPW
> 5 Especially myocarditis but also pericarditis and endocarditis

# Weak left radial pulse

## CATS

| | |
|---|---|
| **C** | **C**oarctation |
| **A** | **A**rterial line/**A**ngiogram[1]/**A**therosclerosis/**A**rteritis[2] |
| **T** | **T**hromboembolism/**T**rauma |
| **S** | **S**ubclavian stenosis[3]/**S**urgery[4] |

1  If entry via radial artery!
2  Especially Takayasu's
3  Often cause by cervical rib
4  Blalock–Taussig shunt: see Fallot's tetralogy (p. 11)

## PACES Causes of a collapsing pulse

### SPLAT

**S**  **S**evere anaemia*
**P**  **P**aget's*/**P**DA (and other large extracardiac shunts)
**L**  **L**oss of conduction tissue (ie complete heart block)
**A**  **A**therosclerosis of the **A**orta/**A**V fistulae
**T**  **T**hyrotoxicosis*

*Splat is the noise made if you imagine the blood collapsing back!
Aortic regurgitation is considered too obvious to mention*

Collapsing pulse = 'hyperdynamic pulse' with a wide pulse pressure

Rarer causes: Wet beri-beri*, $CO_2$ retention and sinus bradycardia

*= High output states

## Part 2 Right-sided aortic arch

### 4 Ts

**T**  **T**etralogy (of Fallot)
**T**  **T**ransposition (of the great arteries)
**T**  **T**runcus arteriosus
**T**  **T**ricuspid atresia

# Left bundle branch block

## CATHOLIC

| | |
|---|---|
| **C** | **C**oronary artery disease |
| **A** | **A**ortic valve disease (especially stenosis) |
| **T** | **T**etralogy of Fallot |
| **H** | **H**ypertension/**H**aemochromatosis/**H**IV |
| **O** | **O**perations to heart |
| **L** | **L**VH |
| **I** | **I**nsertion of RV pacemaker |
| **C** | **C**ardiomyopathy and myocarditis |

*Catholics are known as left-footers!*

# Low voltage ECG

## PITCHS

| | |
|---|---|
| **P** | **P**ericardial effusion: *see* Pericarditis |
| **I** | **I**nfiltrative diseases[1]/**I**nfarction (multiple/global) |
| **T** | $T_4$: low levels of (over and above the effusion it can cause) |
| **C** | **C**OPD/**C**ardiomyopathies |
| **H** | **H**ypopituitarism |
| **S** | **S**evere obesity |

---

**notes**

Incorrect calibration is the other cause

1 Amyloidosis, sarcoidosis, carcinoid or haemochromatosis

# Wolff–Parkinson–White syndrome associations

## Einstein's MATHS

| **Einstein's** | **E**bstein's anomaly[1] |
|---|---|
| **M** | **M**itral valve prolapse |
| **A** | **A**SD |
| **T** | **T**hyrotoxicosis |
| **H** | **H**ypertrophic cardiomyopathy |
| **S** | **S**ex ratio (male:female = 2:1) *Einstein was male!* |

**notes**

Remember to avoid adenosine, digoxin and iv verapamil in this condition. Look for delta wave on ECG (as well as LBBB)

1 Congenital syndrome where the tricuspid valve is displaced into the right ventricle, causing it to become thin and 'atrialised'. Sometimes accompanied by ASD

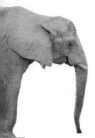

# 3. Respiratory medicine

## Pleural effusion exudate

### PANDA SPRINTS

| | |
|---|---|
| **P** | **P**neumonia[1] |
| **A** | **A**bscess[2]/**A**sbestosis (leads on to neoplasm) |
| **N** | **N**eoplasm[3] |
| **D** | **D**ressler's syndrome[4] |
| **A** | **A**cute rheumatic fever* (and Familial Mediterranean Fever*) |
| **S** | **S**urgery (cardiothoracic) |
| **P** | **P**ancreatitis/**PAN*** |
| **R** | **R**heumatoid arthritis[5]* |
| **I** | **I**nfarction, ie PE[6] |
| **N** | **N**ails: yellow nail syndrome[7] |
| **T** | **T**rauma[8] |
| **S** | **S**LE/**S**cleroderma*/**S**jögren's* |

---

Three Xs:

**X** E**X**udate

**X** E**X**tra – protein (>30 g/l, or fluid:serum ratio >0.5)
- LDH (>200 IU or fluid:serum ratio >0.6)
- $H^+$ (pH <7.1) is suggestive but not necessary!
- Glucose consumption in pneumonias and rheumatoid arthritis

**X** E**X**citing causes: transudates are the more 'boring' causes, ie all the organ failures, plus a few extras – see below

1 Bacterial of course most common (including TB) but remember rarer fungal, parasitic or viral infections

2 Pleural *or subdiaphragmatic* (especially hepatic) abscess when the effusion is a reaction to diaphragmatic inflammation

notes

3 Especially bronchial carcinoma, but also lymphomas and mesothelioma
4 More commonly causes just pericarditis
5 Also ankylosing spondylitis*, dermatomyositis*
6 Can also, more rarely, cause a transudate
7 Yellow nail syndrome: yellow and curved nails associated with lymphoedema, bronchitis, bronchiectasis, sinusitis, nephrotic syndrome and ↓thyroid
8 Haemothorax, chylothorax and rarely ruptured oesophagus

*Pleural effusions are not common for these diseases

## Pleural effusion transudate

## MOPS

| FAILURES: | Heart[1] |
|---|---|
| | Renal[2]* |
| | Liver (cirrhosis*) |
| | Thyroid (ie hypothyroidism) |

| OTHER CAUSES: | **M**eig's syndrome[3] |
|---|---|
| | **O**ther causes of hypoproteinaemia* |
| | **P**E (exudates more common) |
| | **S**arcoid/**S**VC obstruction |

notes

1 NB Pericarditis is another cardiac cause; can also cause ascites if constrictive
2 Nephrotic syndrome and acute glomerulonephritis
3 Pulmonary effusion + ovarian tumour (usually benign fibroma) + ascites

*Many causes occur due to hypoproteinaemia

## Decreased glucose pulmonary effusion

### MEAT

**M**  **M**alignancy
**E**  **E**mpyema
**A**  **A**rthritis (rheumatoid)
**T**  **T**B

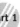 ## Cavitating CXR lesions

 ### TANKS

**Infective**      T      **T**B[1]
    A      **A**spergillosis and other fungi[2]
    N      *N*ocardia
    K      *K*lebsiella
    S      *S*taphylococcus aureus/p*S*eudomonas

**Non-infective**      T      **T**rauma – haematoma
    A      **A**rthritis[3]/**A**NCA (Wegener's)
    N      **N**eoplasms (primary or secondary)
    K      **K**lots, ie PE[4]
    S      **S**arcoid

Other rarer causes:

- Abscesses post chest aspiration/drain (especially if unconscious at time of insertion)
- Hydatid cysts

1  Often calcified and most common in upper lobes
2  Other fungi include histoplasmosis and coccidiomycosis. Often occurs post TB infection (ie fungi grow in 'tuberculous cavity')
3  Rheumatoid nodules – Rheumatoid arthritis or ankylosing spondylitis
4  Especially from infected right heart valves (eg iv lines/drug abuse)

**CXR solitary nodule**

## ABCDEFGHIJ

| | |
|---|---|
| **A** | **A**rtefacts[1] |
| **B** | **B**enign tumours[2] |
| **C** | **C**ancer (including metastases) |
| **D** | **D**ilated bronchus |
| **E** | **E**ffusion[3] |
| **F** | **F**istula (AV) |
| **G** | **G**ranuloma[4] |
| **H** | **H**ydatid cysts |
| **I** | **I**nfections (ie slowly resolving pneumonias) |
| **J** | **J**oint disease (rheumatoid nodules) |

1 Skin lesions, nipples, chest wall abnormalities, ECG or cardiac monitor leads/stickers and buttons or other solid/metallic clothing items
2 Hamartoma, lipomas, adenomas, neurofibromas
3 If interlobar can cause "pseudotumour"
4 TB, sarcoid, histoplasmosis and coccidiomycosis (cat scratch fever)

 **Interstitial lung disease**

 **FIST ACHED**

| | |
|---|---|
| **F** | **F**ungi |
| **I** | **I**diopathic pulmonary fibrosis |
| **S** | **S**arcoid |
| **T** | **T**B/**T**umours |
| | |
| **A** | **A**sbestosis |
| **C** | **C**onnective tissue disease |
| **H** | **H**istiocytosis X[1] |
| **E** | **E**osinophilic granuloma[2]/**E**nvironmental/**E**AA[3] |
| **D** | **D**rugs[4] |

1 See p. 108
2 Autoimmune response to certain infections (especially helminths: see p. 108)
3 Extrinsic allergic alveolitis (= hypersensitivity pneumonitis)
4 See p. 21 for **BBC MANS Gold CAB** (can all cause lower lobe disease)

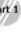

# Upper lobe fibrosis/interstitial shadowing

## HAS PASTE

| | |
|---|---|
| **H** | **H**istoplasmosis |
| **A** | **A**nkylosing spondylitis |
| **S** | **S**ilicosis[1] |
| **P** | **P**neumoconiosis |
| **A** | **A**BPA[2] |
| **S** | **S**arcoid |
| **T** | **T**B |
| **E** | **E**AA[3] |

> **notes**
>
> NB Radiotherapy can cause fibrosis wherever it is applied – look for guidance marks and/or burns on the skin
>
> 1  Can cause progressive massive fibrosis
> 2  Allergic broncho-pulmonary aspergillosis
> 3  Extrinsic allergic alveolitis (= hypersensitivity pneumonitis)

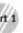

# Lower lobe fibrosis/interstitial shadowing

## BBC MANS Gold CAB

| | |
|---|---|
| **B** | **B**leomycin |
| **B** | **B**usulphan |
| **C** | **C**yclophosphamide |
| **M** | **M**ethotrexate/**M**elphalan |
| **A** | **A**miodarone |
| **N** | **N**itrofurantoin |
| **S** | **S**ulfasalazine |
| **Gold** | Gold |
| **C** | **C**FA[1]/**C**onnective tissue disease[2] |
| **A** | **A**sbestososis |
| **B** | **B**ronchiectasis |

NB Most drugs that cause fibrosis do so in the lower lobe

Radiotherapy can cause fibrosis wherever it is applied – look for guidance marks and/or burns on the skin

1 Cryptogenic fibrosing alveolitis (= idiopathic pulmonary fibrosis): caused by metal, wood, dust, smoke, etc
2 Scleroderma, SLE, dermatomyositis, rheumatoid arthritis. Other rare autoimmune causes are chronic autoimmune hepatitis and ulcerative colitis

 Pneumonia severity assessment

### CURB 65

**British Thoracic Society Guidelines 2004 for community-acquired pneumonia**

**Score 1 point each for:**

C   **C**onfusion[1]
U   **U**rea > 7 mmol/l
R   **R**espiratory rate ≥ 30/min
B   **B**P↓: systolic <90 mmHg **or** diastolic ≤60 mmHg
65   **65** years old (or more)

Score 1 point each for the above 5 features:

- <2: Non-severe; likely suitable for home treatment
- 2: Severe with increased risk of death; consider admission (or hospital-supervised outpatient care) using clinical judgement
- >2: Severe with high risk of death; admit and consider HDU/ITU (especially if ≥4)

1 Abbreviated Mental Test Score ≤8/10 or *new* disorientation in time, place or person

# Clubbing + crackles

## CAB

**C** **C**ryptogenic fibrosing alveolitis
**A** **A**sbestosis (relevant/compatible history?)
**B** **B**ronchiectasis (coarse crackles)/**B**ronchogenic carcinoma (local crackles)

# Adult respiratory distress syndrome

## ARDS ARDS

**A** **A**spiration (and other pneumonias; especially viral)
**R** **R**enal failure
**D** **D**rugs[1]
**S** **S**hock[2]

**A** **A**cute liver failure
**R** **R**aised intracranial pressure
**D** **D**IC/TTP/repeated blood transfusions[3]
**S** **S**moke inhalation[4]

> **notes**
>
> Increased alveolar capillary permeability causes alveolar and interstitial oedema, usually 12–48 h after exposure to cause. When resolves can leave fibrosis
>
> Rarer causes: eclampsia, vasculitis, altitude sickness and near drowning
>
> 1 Salicylates, opiates (especially heroin, diamorphine and methadone), phenobarbital (and other barbiturates) and paraquat
> 2 Sepsis, trauma (including complicated surgery), pancreatitis (acute), severe burns, anaphylaxis/hypersensitivity or prolonged hypotension of any cause
> 3 Other iatrogenic causes: oxygen toxicity, mechanical ventilation, cardiopulmonary bypass, radiation
> 4 Nitrogen dioxide inhalation and other noxious gases can cause this too

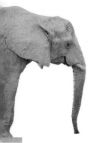

# 4. Gastroenterology

   Hepatomegaly

## 3Cs and 3Is

**C**   **C**hronic liver disease/**C**irrhosis[1]
**C**   **C**ancer ($2° >> 1°$)[2]
**C**   **C**CF

**I**   **I**nfections: hepatitis A/B/C, IMN, hydatid disease
**I**   **I**nflammation: sarcoid/SLE
**I**   **I**nfiltration: amyloid, Gaucher's and other sphingolipidoses

---

**notes**

Other rare conditions: Budd–Chiari syndrome

1 Especially early (liver later shrinks). Causes include: EtOH, primary biliary cirrhosis, haemochromatosis, Wilson's, $\alpha_1$ antitrypsin deficiency, cryptogenic, hepatitis B or C, lupoid, drugs (eg methyldopa/amiodarone/methotrexate)

2 Also remember lymphomas, leukaemias and carcinoid

Remember to look hard for lymphadenopathy and comment on whether it is found when presenting a case. Differential changes and most likely causes now become lymphomas, CLL and IMN

---

## Splenomegaly

### NIHILIST

| | | |
|---|---|---|
| **N** | **N**eoplasm: | Myeloproliferatives[1] |
| | | Lymphoproliferatives[2] |
| **I** | **I**nfection: | Viral: EBV/IMN/glandular fever, hepatitis |
| | | Bacterial (typhoid, brucella, TB) |
| | | Protozoal: malaria*, kala-azar*[3] |
| **H** | **H**aemolytic anaemias: if chronic[4] | |
| **I** | **I**nfiltration: amyloid, lipids (Gaucher's/Niemann Pick) | |
| **L** | **L**iver/**L**iquor[5] | |
| **I** | **I**nflammatory: rheumatoid arthritis[6], SLE, sarcoid | |
| **S** | **S**pherocytosis/**S**BE/**S**lender young females | |
| **T** | **T**rauma/**T**hyrotoxicosis | |

> 1 Myelofibrosis*, CML*, PRV, essential thrombocythemia
> 2 Most lymphomas, CLL, hairy cell leukaemia
> 3 'Black sickness' = visceral infection with *Leishmania donovani*
> 4 For example, autoimmune haemolytic anaemia, cold haemagglutinin, spherocytosis and haemoglobinopathies
> 5 And other causes of portal hypertension: hepatic or portal vein thrombosis, CCF
> 6 If also leucopoenia = Felty's!
>
> *Causes of massive splenomegaly

## Hepatosplenomegaly

### CML III

| | |
|---|---|
| **C** | **C**irrhosis (with portal HTN)/Budd–Chiari[1] |
| **M** | **M**yeloproliferative disorders[2] |
| **L** | **L**ymphoproliferative disorders[3] |
| **I** | **I**nfections: hepatitis, *Brucella*, Weil's, toxoplasmosis, CMV, EBV (IMN) |
| **I** | **I**nflammation: sarcoid, pernicious anaemia |
| **I** | **I**nfiltration: amyloid, Gaucher's and other sphingolipidoses |

> 1 Causes: OCP, tumour, hypercoagulable states, myeloproliferative disorders, hydatid disease, PNH, trauma, radiotherapy
> 2 CML, myelofibrosis, PRV, essential thrombocytopenia ±AML
> 3 CLL, lymphoma, myelomatosis, Waldenstrom's
>
> If lymphadenopathy, lymphoma is most likely but also consider **CHEST**:
>
> **C** **C**LL
> **H** **H**epatitis A, B or C
> **E** **E**BV (ie infective mononucleosis = glandular fever)
> **S** **S**arcoid
> **T** **T**oxoplasmosis

## Ascites

### 5Ps and 5Hs

**P** **P**ortal hypertension (cirrhosis/Budd–Chiari)
**P** **P**eritoneal metastases
**P** **P**eritoneal infection (especially TB)
**P** **P**ericarditis (constrictive)
**P** **P**ancreatitis

**H** **H**eart failure (right-sided or CCF)
**H** **H**epatic failure
**H** **H**ypoalbuminaemia (especially nephrotic syndrome)
**H** **H**ypothyroid
**H** **H**epatic vein thrombosis

NB Similar causes to pleural exudates (see pp. 17–18)

## Primary biliary cirrhosis (Associations/features)

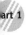

### SCRATCHED

**S** **S**jögren's/**S**cleroderma
**C** **C**oeliac disease
**R** **R**heumatoid arthritis
**A** **A**utoantibodies: '**MSN**'[1]
**T** **T**hyroiditis/**T**ubular acidosis (renal)
**C** **C**opper deposition[2]
**H** **H**LA DR8 (or HLA C4B2)
**E** **E**yes (Kayser–Fleischer rings[2])
**D** **D**ermatomyositis

*Scratch marks are one of the hallmarks of the disease. All causes of cholestasis can lead to pruritus, but in primary biliary cirrhosis it is often the most distressing symptom for patients*

1 **MSN** = **M**itochondrial (95%), **S**mooth muscle (50%), **N**uclear (20%)
2 NB Wilson's is not the only cause of this (see p. 82)

Rx:

- Ursodeoxycholic acid, fat-soluble vitamins and liver transplant
- Consider immunosuppressants: penicillamine (or steroids, azathioprine, methotrexate, ciclosporin A)

 Hepatitis C

 **4Cs**

| | |
|---|---|
| C | **C**hronic |
| C | **C**irrhosis |
| C | **C**ancer |
| C | **C**ryoglobulins (mixed essential type) |

Pancreatitis: modified Glasgow criteria

**GLASGOW Concerns Us**

| | |
|---|---|
| G | **G**eriatric (age >55 years)[1] |
| L | **L**DH >600 IU/l |
| A | **A**lbumin < 32 g/l |
| S | **A**ST >200 IU/l (NB **not** ALT!) |
| G | **G**lucose > 10 mmol/l |
| O | **O**xygen: $PaO_2$ <8 kPa |
| W | **W**hite cells >15·$10^9$/l |
| **C**oncerns | **C**a <2 mmol/l |
| **U**s | **U**rea >16 mmol/l |

GLASGOW Concerns Us lists poor prognostic factors for acute pancreatitis

1 Is not strictly part of Glasgow criteria but is assoc with increased mortality

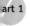

## Gardner's syndrome

### A SOD

**A** **A**denomas of colon[1]/**A**utosomal dominant[2]

Associated with:

**S** **S**ebaceous (or epidermoid) cysts
**O** **O**steomas[3]
**D** **D**ermoid tumours[4]

> **notes**
>
> 1 Polyposis coli: premalignant so careful monitoring ±prophylactic polypectomy or colectomy required
> 2 Chromosome 5
> 3 Of skull: especially mandible and sinuses
> 4 Especially in abdominal wounds (can also get post-op mesenteric fibromatosis)

## (Non-specific) abdominal mass

### CACA CLOT

**C** **C**rohn's
**A** **A**ppendix*
**C** **C**arcinoma (especially ovary or sarcoma)
**A** **A**moebic abscess

**C** **C**arcinoid
**L** **L**ymphoma
**O** **O**vary*
**T** **T**rauma

> **notes**
>
> *Caca clot means any faecal clot, but obviously this is most likely in left iliac fossa*
>
> *These are more 'place specific'

Fat in liver

 **PODGE**

P   **P**regnancy
O   **O**besity[1]
D   **D**iabetes mellitus
G   **G**alactosaemia/**G**lycogen storage disorders
E   **E**tOH

> 1   And counter intuitively can also be caused by starvation/anorexia and total parenteral nutrition
>
> Other causes: hyperlipidaemia (especially hypertriglyceridemia) and drugs such as amiodarone, methotrexate, corticosteroids and oestrogens

 Malabsorption

 **TROPICAL ZOO**

T   **T**ropical sprue
R   **R**adiation
O   **O**perations (small bowel resection)
P   **P**ancreas: cancer or chronic pancreatitis
I   **I**ntestinal lymphangiectasia
C   **C**oeliac/**C**rohn's
A   **A**ntacids (other drugs: neomycin, cholestyramine)
L   **L**actose intolerance/***L**amblia intestinalis*[1]

Z   **Z**ollinger–Ellison syndrome
O   **O**vergrowth of bacteria (folate often normal or increased!)
O   **O**veractive thyroid (Grave's)

> Other causes: Whipples (NB neuro and cardiac involvement – *see* p. 128) and hypogammaglobulinaemia
>
> 1 = *Giardia lamblia*

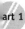
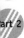

# Toxic megacolon

## BACTERIAS

**B** **B**ehçet's (and Chaga's)
**A** **A**nti-diarrhoea drugs*/**A**ntidepressants*/**A**nticholinergics*
**C** *C*lostridium difficile/**C**MV/*C*ampylobacter (*Yersinia*)
**T** *T*rypanosoma cruzi
**E** *E*ntamoeba histolytica (amoebic dysentery)
**R** **R**adiation (or chemotherapy) colitis
**I** **I**schaemic colitis
**A** **A**nalgesics*/**A**nxiolytics*
**S** *S*almonella (typhoid and non-typhoid)/*S*higella

> **notes**
>
> **Inflammatory bowel disease (IBD) is considered too obvious to mention!**
>
> *Can all increase risk in those with IBD
>
> > ### Diagnosis
> >
> > - Colon >6 cm radiographically
> > - 3 of: (1) fever, (2) tachycardia, (3) ↑WCC, (4) ↓Hb
> > - 1 of: (1) dehydration, (2) altered mental state, (3) electrolyte abnormalities, (4) ↓BP
>
> Is associated with increased colonic wall thickness, multiple air levels and loss of haustral pattern, as seen on abdominal Xray

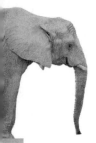

# 5. Endocrinology

art 1
## Addison's disease

art 2
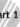
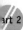

### 17As

| | |
|---|---|
| A | **A**norexia/weight loss |
| A | **A**bdominal pain/vomiting/constipation |
| A | **A**rthralgia/**A**ching muscles[1] |
| A | **A**lopecia |
| A | **A**sthenia (depression/loss of libido) |
| A | **A**lways **A**wake (sleep disorder) |
| A | **A**nxiety |
| A | **A**xillary/**A**nal/**A**reolae/**A**reas of pressure: hyperpigmentation[2] |
| A | **A**rterial hypotension (postural drop) |
| A | **A**naemia[3] |
| A | **A**ldosterone deficiency and excess |
| A | **A**DH $\Rightarrow$ salt/$H_2O$ abnormalities |
| A | **A**CTH test: syn**acth**en |
| A | **A**cidosis |
| A | **A**dditional $K^+$ and $Ca^{++}$ |
| A | **A**bnormal LFTs |
| A | **A**ssociations: |

- **A**trophic gastritis
- **A**nti-21,hydroxylase **A**ntibodies (in 80–90%)
- **A**utoimmune: HLA DR3 B6, **A**drenal **A**ntibodies and other[4]
- **A**drenal infections: **A**cid fast bacilli (ie TB)/**A**IDS[5]

**notes**

Other: hypoglycaemia, loose/damp skin, sunken eyes

1  Are also weak due to salt/$H_2O$ abnormalities
2  Due to ↑**ACTH**. Also see this inside cheeks, in skin creases/scars and sclerae
3  With raised lymphocytes and eosinophils but low neutrophils
4  Grave's, Hashimoto's, diabetes mellitus, pernicious anaemia, hypoparathyroidism and vitiligo
5  eg via CMV, *Mycobacterium avium* infections

**Part 1** Causes of adrenal insufficiency

**6Is**

I   **I**mmune: Addison's*
I   **I**nherited: congenital adrenal hyperplasia, pseudohypoaldosteronism[1] or adrenoleukodystrophy[2]**
I   **I**nfections:
  ● TB*
  ● Meningococcal septicaemia[3]
  ● Viruses**: HIV/CMV
  ● Fungal**: eg histoplasmosis
I   **I**nfiltration:
  ● Metastases** (from lung and breast)
  ● Other: amyloid, sarcoid, haemochromatosis
I   **I**nfarction: especially venous thrombosis after trauma or venography (iatrogenic)
I   **I**atrogenic: ketoconazole, rifampicin, anticoagulants (haemorrhage)

**notes**

1  Pseudohypoaldosteronism: genetic (autosomal dominant or recessive) cause of decreased response of renal tubules to aldosterone
2  Adrenoleukodystrophy: X-linked recessive; long-chain fatty acid esters of cholesterol accumulation. Juvenile-onset (before 12 years old and rapidly progressive) or adult-onset (progressive neurological deficits) forms
3  Causes haemorrhage into adrenals (= Waterhouse–Friderichsen's syndrome)

*Common causes
**Rare causes

## rt 1 Acromegaly

### ABCDEFGHI

| | |
|---|---|
| **A** | **A**rthropathy |
| **B** | **B**P ↑ |
| **C** | **C**arpal tunnel syndrome |
| **D** | **D**iabetes |
| **E** | **E**nlarged tongue, heart and thyroid |
| **F** | **F**ield defects (classically bitemporal hemianopia) |
| **G** | **G**iant hands, feet, frontal bones, cartilage, etc |
| **H** | **H**eadaches[1] |
| **I** | **I**GF-1[2] |

> 1 One of the most common first symptoms (along with sweating)
> 2 Insulin-like growth factor 1 mediates all tissue effects of growth hormone

## rt 1 Thyroid cancer (Types and frequency)

### Popular Foul MEN Live – Arrivederci!

Relative frequency is given in brackets after each type

| | |
|---|---|
| **Popular** | **P**apillary (60% and easily most common) |
| **Foul** | **F**ollicular (25%; poor prognosis) |
| **MEN** | **M**edullary (5%; can be associated with multiple endocrine neoplasia II, as well as familial or sporadic) |
| **Live** | **L**ymphoma (5%; good prognosis) |
| **Arrivederci** | **A**naplastic (<1%; arrivederci = "goodbye" in Italian: worst prognosis!) |

# Hypoglycaemia

## ExPLAIN Malaria

| | |
|---|---|
| **Ex** | **Ex**ogenous drugs: insulin, oral hypoglycaemics and others[1] |
| **P** | **P**ituitary insufficiency |
| **L** | **L**iver failure (+inherited enzyme defects) |
| **A** | **A**ddison's |
| **I** | **I**nsulinoma/**I**mmune[2] |
| **N** | **N**on-pancreatic neoplasms[3] |

**Malaria** Malaria

*Can you explain why malaria is a cause – I can't!*

> 1 EtOH, statins, ACE inhibitors, 4-quinolones
> 2 For example, Hodgkin's ⇒ anti-insulin-receptor antibodies
> 3 Especially retroperitoneal fibrosarcomas and haemangiopericytomas

# Pseudo Cushing's

## PSEUDO

| | |
|---|---|
| **P** | **P**COS |
| **S** | **S**tress |
| **E** | **E**tOH |
| **U** | **U**terus with baby (ie pregnancy!) |
| **D** | **D**epression |
| **O** | **O**besity |

> Looks like Cushing's clinically but isn't
>
> Urinary cortisols, midnight and 9 am cortisols or overnight suppression test may be abnormal (ie raised levels and/or lack of diurnal variation), but will mostly suppress with low-dose dexamethasone suppression test

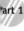

# Polycystic ovary syndrome

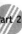

## Male HAIR Increases TLC

| | |
|---|---|
| **Male** | Male pattern baldness |
| **H** | **H**irsutism/**H**eavy (obese) |
| **A** | **A**cne |
| **I** | **I**rregular menstruation |
| **R** | **R**educed fertility |
| **Increases TLC** | Increased levels of **T**estosterone*, **L**H and **C**holesterol |

> **notes**
>
> It is easy to remember to increase TLC (tender loving care) for people suffering from this condition. Insulin levels also go up in response to peripheral resistance. The other hormone abnormalities can be deduced from what has increased, as the similar hormones are decreased, ie oestrogen** and FSH (LH to FSH ratio normally ≥2:1)
>
> *Testosterone not always ↑ (due to ↓ sex hormone binding globulin ↓ing measured levels – no 'free' assay yet available)
> **Oestrogen levels can be hard to intercept as vary widely with menstrual cycle/ovulation

# Multiple endocrine neoplasia (MEN)

### Type I

## PAT Double P

| | |
|---|---|
| **P** | **P**arathyroid: adenomas (95% exhibit hyperparathyroidism) |
| **A** | **A**drenal: adenoma (non-functioning) |
| **T** | **T**hyroid: adenoma (multiple or single) |
| **P** | **P**ituitary: prolactinoma, Cushing's (disease), acromegaly |
| **P** | **P**ancreas: insulinoma, glucagonoma, gastrinoma or VIPoma[1] |

### Type IIa

## PAT (No Ps)

| | |
|---|---|
| **P** | **P**arathyroid: adenomas (20% exhibit hyperparathyroidism) |
| **A** | **A**drenal: phaeochromocytoma or adenoma (causing Cushing's syndrome) |
| **T** | **T**hyroid (cancers – especially medullary) |

**Type IIb** As type IIa but never hyperparathyroidism and also has the following:

- Marfanoid body habitus
- Ganlioneuroma: visceral (especially GI)
- Neuromas: especially lips and tongue

**notes**

### Type I

- Affects the greater number of endocrine tissues
- All are autosomal dominant

1  VIP = Vasoactive intestinal polypeptide: a GI neuropeptide that increases secretions. In excess it causes watery diarrhoea and decreased K and Cl

### Type IIa

- Affects a smaller number of tissues but has more substantial clinical effects (ie functioning adenomas or carcinomas)
- Are all caused by the 'RET' proto-oncogene (on chromosome 10 – screen relatives for thyroid cancer!)

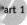

# Types of diabetic neuropathy

## GAMA

**G** **G**love and stocking[1]
**A** **A**utonomic[2]
**M** **M**ononeuritis multiplex[3]
**A** **A**myotrophy[4]

1 'Classical' peripheral neuropathy (see p. 69) – often painful
2 Autonomic neuropathy: 40% of diabetics have detectable autonomic dysfunction but a few are symptomatic: *postural hypotension, neuropathic bladder* (incomplete emptying ±overflow incontinence or UTIs), *bowel dysfunction* (gastric stasis with diarrhoea – especially at night – or constipation) and *sexual dysfunction* (erectile and/or ejaculatory failure – note vascular disease and depression also contribute)
3 Especially cranial nerves III, IV, VI and median, ulnar and lateral popliteal nerves
4 Amyotrophy:
   - Motor polyneuropathy – is normally asymmetrical and classically causes proximal weakness (lower limbs more common than upper)
   - Is thought to be due to vascular damage to large nerve trunks or roots
   - As with all lower motor neurone conditions reflexes are diminished and wasting is seen in affected areas although interestingly extensor plantars can be seen
   - Sensory loss can also be seen (especially in the thigh) and can also cause severe pain (especially at night) and is often the cause of presentation
   - Recovery normally occurs with restoration of good control of blood sugar

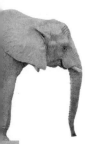

# 6. Metabolic medicine

## Disproportionate rise of creatinine or urea

**RHABDO GASTRO**

### CREATININE > UREA

| | |
|---|---|
| R | **RHABDO**myolysis |
| H | **H**epatic failure |
| A | **A**ntibiotics, especially trimethoprim/septrin[1] |
| B | **B**lack ethnic groups (African Caribbean) |
| D | **D**ialysis patients |
| O | **O**ther: low protein intake |

### UREA > CREATININE

| | |
|---|---|
| G | **GASTRO**intestinal bleed[2] |
| A | **A**trophied muscles[3] |
| S | **S**tasis (of urine) |
| T | **T**etracyclines[4] |
| R | **R**enal failure |
| O | **O**ther: dehydration |

*Most common cause of each is the first listed (and therefore is also the actual mnemonic)*

---

**notes**

1 Note tetracyclines do the opposite!
2 And other causes of high protein load
3 Including muscle wasting, cachexia and catabolic states
4 Note trimethoprim/septrin do the opposite!

---

# Hyperkalaemia

## 'Additional'

| | |
|---|---|
| **A** | **A**dded $K^+$: iatrogenic iv fluids (incl. transfusions)/ po supplements |
| **A** | **A**cidosis – **A**cute renal failure, DKA, RTA |
| **A** | **A**ddison's |
| **A** | **A**miloride (+ other K-sparing drugs) |
| **A** | **A**CE inhibitors/**A**ngiotensin receptor blockers |
| **A** | **A**naesthetics (suxamethonium) |
| **A** | **A**nti-tumour agents (cause cell lysis) |
| **A** | **A**noxia/tissue damage |
| **A** | N**a** depletion |
| **A** | **A**rtefactual (haemolysis) |

# MRCP-level causes of hypokalaemia

## ADD POTASSIUM if ILL

| | |
|---|---|
| **A** | **A**lkalosis/**A**ccelerated hypertension* |
| **D** | **D**iuretics* |
| **D** | **D**iarrhoea |
| **P** | **P**eriodic paralysis |
| **O** | **O**ral loss (vomiting!) |
| **T** | **T**ubular disorders[1] |
| **A** | **A**ldosterone-producing tumour (Conn's) |
| **S** | **S**tenosis of renal artery* |
| **S** | **S**tarvation (including anorexia) |
| **I** | **I**leostomy |
| **U** | **U**terosigmoidoscopy |
| **M** | **Mg**, milk of |

(if)

| | |
|---|---|
| **I** | **I**nsulin |
| **L** | **L**iver cirrhosis with ascites* |
| **L** | **L**eukaemia (+ lysozymuria due to muramidase production) |

notes

1 Tubular disorders:

- Renal tubular acidosis (RTA)
- Nephrotic syndrome
- Liddle's syndrome: inherited disorder causing increased distal tubular retention of Na but loss of K; also causes $\downarrow\downarrow$ aldosterone levels; causes hypertension and alkalosis; treatment: triamterene
- Bartter's syndrome: $\downarrow$ renotubular reabsorption of Na $\Rightarrow$ $\uparrow$ K, Na and Cl excreted in urine; also $\uparrow$ renal synthesis of prostaglandins $\Rightarrow$ $\uparrow$ renin $\Rightarrow$ $\uparrow$ aldosterone; also $\uparrow$ $HCO_3$; Diagnosis: renal biopsy (hyperplasia of juxtaglomerular apparatus), $\uparrow$ urinary prostaglandin excretion (and $\downarrow$ responsiveness of vasculature to pressor effects of angiotensin II, therefore BP stays normal). NB Can be mimicked by diuretic abuse clinically. Treatment: indometacin

*Occur via secondary hyperaldosteronism

## Hypercalcaemia

### SUPRA ACTIVE PTH

| | |
|---|---|
| **S** | **S**arcoid |
| **U** | **U**raemia |
| **P** | **P**aget's (if immobile) |
| **R** | **R**enal failure (secondary and tertiary $\uparrow$ PTH) |
| **A** | **A**ddison's |

| | |
|---|---|
| **A** | **A**rtificial ("cuffed" sample?) |
| **C** | **C**ancer*: via bone metastases/PTH-related peptide[1] |
| **T** | **T**hiazides |
| **I** | **I**mmobilisation |
| **V** | **V**itamin D (or A) toxicity |
| **E** | **E** prostaglandins |

| | |
|---|---|
| **P** | **P**lasma cells (= multiple myeloma!) |
| **T** | **T**hyrotoxicosis/**T**B |
| **H** | **H**yperparathyroidism (primary)** |

notes

1 Paraneoplastic syndrome: produced by kidney, lung or ovarian tumours

*Causes half of all cases
**Other common cause: primary, secondary or tertiary

Other rare causes: berylliosis or lithium

# Metabolic acidosis

## LUKE'S GREAT PAL

### Increased anion gap $(Na^+ + K^+) - (HCO_3^- + Cl^-) > 16$ mmol/l

**L**  **L**actate[1]
**U**  **U**rea: RF
**K**  **K**etones: DKA, starvation
**E**  **E**thylene glycol (antifreeze)
**S**  **S**alicylates

### Normal anion gap $(Na^+ + K^+) - (HCO_3^- + Cl^-) = 12–16$ mmol/l

**G**  **G**I causes[2]
**R**  **R**enal failure
**E**  Chol**E**styramine
**A**  **A**cetazolamide (Carbonic anhydrase inhibitors)
**T**  **T**ubular acidosis

### Reduced anion gap $(Na^+ + K^+) - (HCO_3^- + Cl^-) = <12$ mmol/l

**P**  **P**lasma cells (= multiple myeloma)
**A**  **A**lbumin loss (ie nephrotic syndrome)
**L**  **L**ithium

---

1  Types A and B
   - Type **A**: ↑**A**naerobic respiration – **A**noxia (including shock, ie tissue anoxia)
   - Type **B**:
     - ↓ **B**reakdown – **B**iguanides (metformin), **B**ooze (including methanol), cyanide, CO, isoniazid
     - ↑ Hepatic production – liver disease, mitochondrial diseases, G6PD deficiency, leukaemias
2  Pancreatic, biliary and other fistulae, uretosigmoidoscopy, severe diarrhoea

# Metabolic alkalosis

## VOMED

**V** **V**omiting[1] or aspiration

**O** **O**vercorrection of chronic $\uparrow CO_2$ or any acidosis

**M** **M**ineralocorticoid excess[2]

**E** **E**thylene glycol poisoning/**E**arly Sepsis

**D** **D**iuretics[3]/**D**iarrhoea (Cl-losing)

> Other: Ingestion of alkali (rare!) or excessive antacids (again rare!)
>
> 1 Especially pyloric stenosis
> 2 Cushing's, Conn's or carbenoxolone poisoning
> 3 And other decreased-$K^+$ states which increase renal $H^+$ loss by distal convoluted tubule

# Respiratory acidosis

## OH NO DR T!

**O** **O**bstructive of airways: COPD and asthma (acute) or aspiration

**H** **H**ypoventilation

**N** **N**euromuscular[1]

**O** **O**besity

**D** **Drugs**: anaesthetics and other sedatives

**R** **Respiratory** disease: fibrosis, severe pneumonia, ARDS

**T** **T**horacic cage deformities[2]

> 1 Especially Guillain–Barré, polio, motor neurone disease, cerebral trauma/tumour and neurotoxins (tetanus, botulism, curare)
> 2 Especially flail chest and severe kyphoscoliosis

Part 1 Respiratory alkalosis

 Part 2 **CHOPPA**

C **C**erebral[1]
H **H**ypoxia[2]/**H**epatic failure
O **O**verventilation (mechanical)[3]
P **P**ulmonary disease (PE or pulmonary oedema)
P **P**sychological (hysteria/stress/pain)
A **A**spirin toxicity

> **notes**
> 1 Trauma, tumour or infection (also Gram-negative sepsis)
> 2 High altitude, severe anaemia and pulmonary disease
> 3 If on ITU or during anaesthesia

 Part 1 Pellagra

 Part 2 **5Ds**

D **D**ermatitis (photosensitive)
D **D**ementia
D **D**iarrhoea
D **D**epression
D **D**eath

> **notes**
> - Caused by niacin (= nicotinamide) deficiency
> - Also causes loss of appetite, neurological features (weakness, neuropathy, tremor, ataxia, rigidity and fits) and glossitis/stomatitis
> - Seen if severely malnourished (especially if maize is a major constituent of diet, in carcinoid syndrome and Hartnup disease)

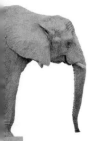

# 7. Renal medicine

## Chronic renal failure

### 6Ps

| | |
|---|---|
| P | **P**ulmonary oedema[1] |
| P | **P**ericarditis |
| P | **P**eripheral neuropathy |
| P | **P**ruritus |
| P | **P**igmentation |
| P | **P**arathyroid overactivity |

> 1 Can be acute on chronic presentation as 'flash pulmonary oedema'

## Papillary necrosis

### POSTCARD

| | |
|---|---|
| P | **P**yelonephritis |
| O | **O**bstruction |
| S | **S**ickle |
| T | **T**B |
| C | **C**irrhosis/**C**oagulopathy |
| A | **A**nalgesic nephropathy (**A**spirin/NSAIDs) |
| R | **R**enal vein thrombosis |
| D | **D**iabetes mellitus |

**Part 1** Interstitial nephritis

 **Part 2** Drugs

### SLAPPERS Misuse Diuretics and CIPRO

| | |
|---|---|
| S | **S**alicylates (+ other NSAIDS) |
| L | **L**ead |
| A | **A**llopurinol |
| P | **P**henindione |
| P | **P**enicillin (+ β lactams) |
| E | **E**thambutol |
| R | **R**ifampicin |
| S | **S**ulphonamides |

| | |
|---|---|
| **Mi**suse | **M**ethyldopa |

| | |
|---|---|
| **Diuretics**: | Thiazides/frusemide |

| | |
|---|---|
| C | **C**iprofloxacin |
| I | **I**soniazid |
| P | **P**enicillin |
| R | **R**ifampicin |
| O | Sulph**O**namides |

### Other

### LEPRO

| | |
|---|---|
| L | **Lepto**spirosis |
| E | **E**BV |
| P | **P**arvovirus |
| T | **T** cell deficiency (ie HIV) |
| O | **O**ther: sickle |

 **Part 1** Alport's

**Part 2** SEX

| | |
|---|---|
| S | **S**ensorineural deafness (bilateral) |
| E | **E**nd-stage renal failure[1]/**E**ye abnormalities[2] |
| X | **X**-linked[3] |

*SEX-linked, ie X linked!*

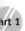

Can also cause hypertension and UTIs

1 Haematuria (microscopic) and proteinuria
2 Cataracts, macular lesions and anterior lenticonus (protrusion of lens into anterior chamber)
3 Usually dominant (rarely recessive) defect of type IV collagen gene, causing basement membrane abnormalities, which in the glomerulus leads to thickening of this membrane. Carrier females may have urinary abnormalities but most don't develop renal failure

# Indications for urgent dialysis in ARF

## 4Ps

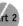

P **P**otassium > 6.5 mmol/l[1] (or lower if ECG changes)
P **P**H < 7.1
P **P**ulmonary oedema[2]
P **P**ericarditis[3]

NB: dialysis is normally only indicated for the first 3 in this list if are refractory to other (1st line) treatments. Other indications is very severe uraemia: eg urea >60 mmol/l or symptoms such as encephalopathy or intractable vomiting

1 Or lower if ECG changes
2 Unresponsive to other treatment
3 Not due to other causes

# False-positive Clinistix®

## ACIDS

A **A**spirin
C **C** vitamin (ascorbic acid)
I **I**nky ears: alkaptonuria[1]
D **D**iabetes mellitus (glucose)
S **S**ugars (other than glucose): fructose, pentose, lactose

NB *Are not false-positive for clini**test** sticks*

1 Alkaptonuria = ochronosis: homogentisic acid deficiency. Pigment accumulates in cartilage (can see dark discoloration, especially in ears and sclera) and causes arthritis, especially knees and back. Causes secondary calcification in joints that is seen on radiography. Treatment: low protein diet

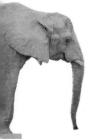

# 8. Rheumatology

## Seronegative arthritides

### CRAP

C   **C**rohn's/UC
R   **R**eiter's
A   **A**nkylosing spondylitis
P   **P**soriatic arthritis

> **notes**
>
> Seronegativity means rheumatoid-factor-negative. All these conditions are linked by strong association with HLA-B27 and development of spondylitis + sacroiliitis
>
> Whipple's disease (see p. 128) and Behçet's are sometimes also considered part of this group

## Anaemia in rheumatoid arthritis

### CAMP Gold Felt

C       **C**hronic disease: anaemia of
A       **A**spirin[1]
M       **M**ethotrexate (**M**egaloblastic[2])
P       **P**ernicious anaemia (if associated)

**Gold**    Gold (via bone marrow suppression[3])

**Felt**    Felty's[4]

notes

1 Plus other NSAIDs: causes iron deficiency anaemia
2 Via folate deficiency
3 Also caused by indomethacin, penicillamine
4 Felty's: rheumatoid arthritis + splenomegaly/lymphadenopathy + blood disorder (neutropenia, thrombocytopenia and anaemia). Can cause recurrent infections

## Rheumatoid lung

### NAPE

N   **N**odules[1]
A   **A**lveolitis/fibrosis
P   **P**leurisy/**P**neumoconiosis[2]
E   **E**ffusion

notes

Other rarer features are cricoarytenoid inflammation and obliterative bronchiolitis

1 Almost exclusively occur in rheumatoid-factor-positive patients
2 Caplan's syndrome: large (0.5–2 cm) nodule formation and fibrosis. Treat with steroids

## Ankylosing spondylitis

### 12 As

A   **A**pical fibrosis
A   **A**nterior uveitis[1]
A   **A**ortic regurgitation
A   **A**ortitis
A   **A**V block
A   **A**tlantoaxial subluxation
A   **A**myloidosis
A   **A**chilles tendonitis
A   Ig**A** nephropathy
A   Plantar f**A**sciitis
A   **A**rthritis[2]
A   **A**rachnoiditis (spinal)

> 1 Especially common if there is peripheral joint involvement
> 2 Mostly sacroiliac and axial joints but can also occur peripherally

## SLE lung manifestations

### CHEST

| | |
|---|---|
| **C** | **C**rackles: interstitial pneumonia ±basal atelectasis |
| **H** | **H**aemorrhage (vasculitis) |
| **E** | **E**ffusions ±pleurisy |
| **S** | **S**hrunken lung – diaphragmatic myopathy |
| **T** | **T**B (and other pneumonias) |

## Behçet's

### ULCER

| | |
|---|---|
| **U** | **U**lcers: oral*(100%) genital* (80%)/**U**veitis*[1] |
| **L** | **L**arge joint asymmetrical polyarthropathy[2] |
| **C** | **C**NS lesions[3]/**C**olchicine treatment/**C**iclosporin treatment (especially for eyes) |
| **E** | **E**mbolism (thrombophlebitis)/**E**rythema nodosum/**E**nteral involvement[4] |
| **R** | **R**ash[5] |

> 1 Can also get 'vascular eye' – can cause blindness!***
> 2 Non-erosive and mostly lower limb
> 3 Aseptic meningitis, ataxia, pseudobulbar palsy, TIA-like episodes
> 4 UC-like picture
> 5 Photosensitivity, pathergy**, pustules (spontaneous), vasculitis, folliculitis
>
> *Classical triad
> **Pathergy: pustules at site of trivial injury, eg venepuncture
>
> HLA-B5 association (plus B51 for eyes and B12 for oral ulcers)
> Males as common but more severe
>
> > **Treatment**
> >
> > Systemic **C**orticosteroids or **C**olchicines (**C**iclosporin can be given to save sight)***

**Part 1** Reiter's syndrome (features of)

 **Part 2** **ACUPUNCTure**

| | |
|---|---|
| **A** | **A**rthritis[1]* |
| **C** | **C**onjunctivitis[2]* |
| **U** | **U**rethritis* (generally mild) |
| **P** | **P**lantar fasciitis/Keratoderma blenorrhagica |
| **U** | **U**lcers: oral (painless[3]) |
| **N** | **N**euro involvement[4] |
| **C** | **C**ircinate balanitis |
| **T** | **T**endonitis (especially Achilles) |

**notes**

1 Asymmetrical and mostly lower limb – especially sacroiliitis
2 Often go on later to develop uveitis
3 NB Ulcer can be painful in Behçet's
4 Mostly peripheral neuropathy but CNS involvement can occur

*Form classical triad (rest of symptoms uncommon)

> **Causes**
>
> - Often occurs 1–4 weeks post infections
> - **G**onococcal infections (ie *Neisseria gonorrhoea*) and other (sexually transmitted) urethritis
> - **G**I infections (*Salmonella, Shigella, Yersinia* and *Campylobacter*)
> - Strong HLA-B27 association (as with all seronegative arthritides)

 **Part 1** Antiphospholipid syndrome

 **Part 2** **9As**

| | |
|---|---|
| **A** | **A**ntiphospholipid antibodies |
| **A** | **A**PTT increase (and minor PT increase)[1] |
| **A** | **A**nticoagulant (lupus)[2] |
| **A** | **A**nticardiolipin antibodies |
| **A** | **A**rterial (+venous) thrombosis |
| **A** | **A**bortions – recurrent |
| **A** | **A**bnormal behaviour (encephalitis) |
| **A** | **A**rtificially (false) positive VDRL |
| **A** | **A**nticoagulants (warfarin) are drug of choice |

> **notes**
> 1 Fails to correct with plasma treatment (note platelets can decrease)
> 2 Despite being a thrombotic disease there is a paradoxical increase in clotting times in vitro

## Jaccoud's arthropathy

### PURSES

**P** **P**arkinson's is associated
**U** **U**rticarial vasculitis is associated
**R** **R**heumatic fever can cause it
**S** **S**LE (50% of) can cause it
**E** **E**rosions on X-ray (none!!!!)
**S** **S**ubluxation (lots!!!!)

> **notes**
> Reducible, non-erosive deformities of hand joints with a preservation of function: results from tendon inflammation and shortening

## Charcot's joints (causes)

### 4Ss

**S** **S**ugar: diabetes[1]
**S** **S**yphilis[2]
**S** **S**yringomyelia[3]
**S** **S**egregated **S**ocieties = leper colonies, ie *Mycobacterium leprae*!

**Less common causes:**

### 6Ss

**S** **S**pina bifida
**S** **S**pirits (EtOH)
**S** **S**teroid intra-articular injections (multiple)
**S** **S**ubacute combined degeneration of the cord
**S** **S**pastic paraplegia[4]
**S** **S**ensory neuropathies: other, eg HSMN

> **notes**
>
> Charcot's joints (aka neuropathic arthropathies) are caused by loss sensation in the affected limb (especially pain perception) leading to painless destruction of the joint via constant trauma and incomplete repair. Eventually the joint becomes swollen/deformed with new bone formation and features of osteoarthrosis. Range of movement is also affected. Can flare up quickly and mimic septic arthritis, especially in diabetes mellitus
>
> 1 Mostly in feet (especially toes)
> 2 Tabes dorsalis: mostly lower limb (especially knee but also up to lumber vertebrae and down to ankle)
> 3 Syrinx = tubular cavity (CSF filled). These can be found in 'myelia' (cord) or in the 'bulb' (midbrain – looks like a bulb/bulge). Accordingly syringomyelia mostly affects neck/proximal upper limb joints (cervical vertebrae, shoulder and elbow)
> 4 Hips especially affected

 **Part 1** Polyarteritis nodosa (PAN)

 **Part 2** American College of Rheumatology (ACR) criteria

For diagnosis ≥3 of these 10 needed; sensitivity 82% and specificity 87% (Lightfoot RW Jr et al. *Arthritis Rheum* 1990; **33**: 1088–1093)

### WE RANK MAN*

**Testicular T**esticular tenderness[1]

**W** **W**eight loss ≥4 kg since illness began
**E** **E**levated blood pressure: diastolic >90 mmHg

**R** **R**eticular (= 'mottled' or 'net like') **R**ash = livedo reticularis
**A** **A**ntibodies to hepatitis B surface antigen
**N** **N**eutrophils (polymorphonuclear) in biopsy samples of artery wall
**K** **K**idney failure[2]

**M** **M**yalgia, weakness or leg tenderness[3]
**A** **A**rteriographic (angiogram) abnormalities[4]
**N** **N**europathy[5]

notes

*WE RANK MAN can be rearranged into another, somewhat more memorable, mnemonic that reminds you of ANCA[6] and Testicular pain!*

1 Not due to infection, trauma or other causes
2 Raised urea (>40 mg/dl) or creatinine (>150 μmol/l) not due to dehydration or obstruction
3 Diffuse myalgias (excluding shoulder and hip girdle) or weakness of muscles or tenderness of leg muscles
4 Aneurysms or occlusions of the visceral arteries (especially renal but also liver and intestinal arteries), not due to arteriosclerosis, fibromuscular dysplasia or other inflammatory causes
5 Mononeuropathy, mononeuritis multiplex or polyneuropathy
6 cANCA-positive (males>females): microscopic polyarteritis is another cause of cANCA positivity, but Wegener's of course is the most common

### Diagnosis

● Suspect this condition in anyone with major organ disease plus hypertension

### Differential diagnosis

● Polymyalgia rheumatica: has no neuropathy, testicular pain, livedo or immune features

## Henoch–Schonlein purpura

## American College of Rheumatology (ACR) criteria

For diagnosis ≥2 of these 4 needed; sensitivity 87% and specificity 88% (Mills JA et al. *Arthritis Rheum* 1990; **33**: 1114–1121)

### PAGE

| | |
|---|---|
| **P** | **P**alpable **P**urpura[1] |
| **A** | **A**ge ≤ 20 years at onset of symptoms |
| **G** | **G**ranulocytes in walls of arterioles or venules (on biopsy) |
| **E** | **E**nteral angina[2] |

notes

1 Slightly raised palpable haemorrhagic skin lesions, not related to thrombocytopenia
2 Diffuse abdominal pain (worse after meals) or a diagnosis of bowel ischaemia (usually including bloody diarrhoea)

**Part 1** Takayasu's arteritis

**Part 2** American College of Rheumatology (ACR) criteria

For diagnosis ≥3 of these 6 needed; sensitivity 90% and specificity 98%

### CLAUDE

| | |
|---|---|
| **C** | **C**laudication of extremities |
| **L** | **L**ower BP (<10 mmHg) in affected arm |
| **A** | **A**rteriographic (angiogram) abnormality[1] |
| **U** | **U**nder 40 years old |
| **D** | **D**ecreased pulsation of one or both brachial arteries |
| **E** | **E**xcessive noise over one or both subclavian arteries or abdominal aorta ie bruits |

*The name Claude should trigger the main symptom of claudication!*

---

**notes**

1 Narrowing or occlusion of entire aorta, its primary branches, or large arteries in the proximal upper or lower extremities (not due to atherosclerosis, fibromuscular dysplasia or other causes)

Changes are usually focal or segmental

---

**Part 1** SLE diagnostic features

**Part 2** American College of Rheumatology (ACR) criteria

For diagnosis ≥4 of the 11 (serially or simultaneously) are needed during any interval

### MD SOAP BRAIN

| | |
|---|---|
| **M** | **M**alar rash[1] |
| **D** | **D**iscoid rash[2] |
| **S** | **S**erositis: pleuritis[3] or pericarditis[4] |
| **O** | **O**ral (or nasopharyngeal) ulcers: usually painless |
| **A** | **A**rthritis[5] |
| **P** | **P**hotosensitive rash |

**B** **B**lood disorder[6]
**R** **R**enal disorder[7]
**A** **A**NA (antinuclear antibodies)[8]
**I** **I**mmune disorder[9]
**N** **N**euro disorder[10]

> **notes**
>
> 1 Fixed erythema, flat or raised – tending to spare nasolabial folds
> 2 Erythematous, raised patches with adherent keratotic scaling and follicular plugging; atrophic scarring may occur in older lesions
> 3 Pleuritis defined as history of pleuritic pain or rubbing heard by a physician or evidence of pleural effusion
> 4 Pericarditis defined as: ECG evidence or rub or evidence of pericardial effusion
> 5 Tenderness, swelling, or effusion of ≥2 peripheral joints (non erosive!)
> 6 Haemolytic anaemia, leucopoenia, lymphopenia or thrombocytopenia
> 7 Cellular casts/persistent proteinuria (glomerulonephritis: most types can occur)
> 8 ↑ titre ⇒ ↑ positive predictive value
> 9 Anti-DNA antibodies, anti-Sm antibodies, or antiphospholipid antibodies (anticardiolipin antibodies, lupus anticoagulant or false-positive syphilis serology)
> 10 Seizures or psychosis without drug/metabolic cause (eg uraemia, ketoacidosis and electrolyte disturbance)

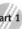

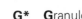

## Wegener's granulomatosis

### GRANULOMAS

**G\*** **G**ranulomatous inflammation on biopsy[1]
**R** **R**ash[2]: vasculitic/purpuric
**A\*** **A**bnormal CXR[3] (nodules, fixed infiltrates or cavities)
**N\*** **N**asal or oral inflammation[4]
**U\*** **U**rinary sediment[5]
**L** **L**oss of hearing: sensorineural and conductive can occur
**O** **O**cular disorders: '**PUS**' **P**roptosis[6], **U**veitis or **S**cleritis
**M** **M**ononeuritis multiplex[7] (cranial or peripheral)/**M**yocarditis (or more commonly pericarditis[8])
**A** **A**NCA: +ve cANCA (cytoplasmic anti-proteinase 3) in 90% of *active* cases/**A**rthritis
**S** **S**ystemic upset: malaise, weight loss, fevers (especially nocturnal – often low grade) and ↑ESR

*Wegener's causes necrotising granulomas of small/medium-sized blood vessels (⇒ vasculitis): if full mnemonic cannot be learnt due to lack of time/brain space focus on 'GRANU'*!*

*The four criteria of the American College of Rheumatology (ACR): ≥2 needed for diagnosis (sensitivity 88%, specificity 92%) (Leavitt RY et al. *Arthritis Rheum* 1990; **33**: 1101–1107)

1  Granulomas are within the wall of the artery or in perivascular or extravascular areas (artery or arteriole)
2  Often with 'migratory pattern': over time lesions clear from one area and appear in another. Also causes nailfold infarcts (and rarely pyoderma gangrenosum see p. 67)
3  Showing presence of nodules, fixed infiltrates or cavities
4  Painful or painless ulcers or purulent/bloody nasal discharge. Can cause nasal bridge collapse ('saddle nose') or haemoptysis
5  Microhaematuria (>5 RBC/high-power field) or RBC casts on microscopy. Focal proliferative glomerulonephritis (±segmental necrosis) is predominant pathology
6  Proptosis = 'Pseudotumour' (retro-orbital infiltration with granulomas)
7  See pp. 72–73. Although mononeuritis multiplex is commonest neurological manifestation intracerebral granulomas can occur making almost any neuro (and even psychiatric) presentation possible
8  Cardiac involvement can also cause arrhythmias

**Treatment**

- Cyclophosphamide and steroids (can enable long-term remission in 90%); untreated survival = 5 months

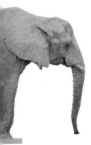

# 9. Dermatology

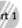
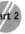

## Erythema nodosum

### SPLOTCHY TIBIALS
S    **S**arcoid/**S**treptococcal infections[1]
P    **P**enicillin/**P**sittacosis/**P**regnancy/**P**ost-radiation therapy
L    **L**ymphoma/**L**eukaemia
O    **O**CP
T    **T**B/BCG vaccination
C    *Chlamydia*/**C**at scratch fever[2]
H    **H**istoplasmosis
Y    *Yersinia*

T    **T**inea (especially *Trichophyton* species)
I    **I**nflammatory bowel disease
B    **B**ehçet's/*Brucella*
I    $I_2/Br_2$ poisoning
A    **A**rteritis (PAN)
L    **L**eprosy/*Lymphogranuloma venereum*/**L**eptospirosis
S    **S**ulphonamides/*Salmonella*

> **notes**
> 1  Sarcoid and streptococcal infections are the most common causes in the UK
> 2  Cat scratch fever = coccidiomycosis (*Bartonella henselae* infection)

## Erythema multiforme

| **DRUGS** | **S** | **S**ulphonamides/**S**ulphonylureas |
| | **P** | **P**enicillin |
| | **O** | **O**CP (and pregnancy) |
| | **Q** | **Q**uinine (antimalarials) |
| **BUGS** | **S** | **S**treptococcal: second commonest |
| | **H** | **H**SV (especially if recurrent): commonest |
| | **O** | **O**rf (Pox virus causing periungual infection) |
| | **T** | **T**B (*Mycobacterium* – also *Mycoplasma*!) |
| **AUTOIMMUNE** | **S** | **S**LE |
| | **P** | **P**AN |
| | **U** | **U**C/Crohn's |
| | **D** | **D**ermatomyositis |
| **CANCERS** | **S** | **S**olid tumours |
| | **L** | **L**ymphoma |
| | **M** | **M**yeloma |

**Idiopathic = 50%!!!!!!!!**

## Psoriasis exacerbation

### STREP

**S**  **STREP**tococcal infections[1]
**T**  **T**rauma
**R**  **R**etroviral (HIV)
**E**  **E**ndocrine (hormones – especially post partum)
**P**  **P**rednisolone withdrawal[2]

> **notes**
> 1 Especially likely to worsen guttate psoriasis
> 2 Or stopping of any other steroid. Other drugs: beta-blockers, lithium, antimalarials

**rt 1** Purpura

**CES** **ARS SPOTS PURPLE**

- **A** **A**ge/**A**nticoagulants
- **R** **R**heumatoid arthritis[1]
- **S** **S**teroids

- **S** **S**epsis
- **P** **P**AN
- **O** **O**sler–Weber–Rendu (HHT)
- **T** **T**hrombocytopenia
- **S** **S**curvy/**S**tasis of veins

- **P** **P**NH
- **U** **U**raemia
- **R** **R**ubella
- **P** **P**araprotein (myeloma)
- **L** **L**upus
- **E** **E**hlers–Danlos

> 1 Phenylbutazone/gold therapy
>
> Other drugs: thiazides, sulphonamides, sulphonylureas, barbiturates

**rt 1** Lichen planus

**ACES**
 **Causes**

**PAM has Lichen Planus**

- **P** **P**enicillin/**P**enicillamine
- **A** **A**u (gold)/**A**rsenic
- **M** **M**ethyldopa
- **L** **L**upus
- **P** **P**henothiazines

**Non-dermatology features**

- **O** **O**ral lesions[1]
- **N** **N**ails can be involved[2]
- **A** **A**lopecia ('cicatricial')[3]

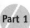

A raised purplish, polygonal rash with flat-topped, shiny and extremely itchy lesions; flexural surfaces (especially wrists) affected most

1  Can rarely lead to squamous cell carcinoma. Can often see 'Wickham's striae' (white lacy pattern) on surface of lesions
2  Longitudinal thinning or loss of whole nail
3  Occurs occasionally in patches (permanent)

---

**Part 1**  # Erythroderma causes

## I'D SCALP

| | |
|---|---|
| **I** | **I**diopathic (30%) |
| **D** | **D**rugs (28%): most commonly used drugs can cause this! |
| **S** | **S**eborrhoeic dermatitis |
| **C** | **C**ontact dermatitis |
| **A** | **A**topic dermatitis |
| **L** | **L**ymphoma/**L**eukaemia |
| **P** | **P**soriasis |

Aka Generalised exfoliative dermatitis

Definition: >90% of skin surface area involved

Complications: infections/sepsis, hypoalbuminaemia, high output cardiac failure, ↓ thermoregulation

---

**Part 1**  # Vitiligo associations

## Pale Pigmentation PATCH

| | |
|---|---|
| **Pale** | **P**ernicious anaemia |

**Pigmentation**  **P**BC

| | |
|---|---|
| **P** | **P**remature ovarian failure/**P**roliferative glomerulonephritis |
| **A** | **A**ddison's/**A**trophic gastritis/**A**lopecia areata/Ig **A** nephritis |
| **T** | **T**hyroid disease (Grave's or Hashimoto's) |
| **C** | **C**AH/**C**andidiasis/**C**oeliac disease/**C**FA |
| **H** | **H**ypoparathyroidism (idiopathic)/**H**ypergammaglobulinaemia |

# Hyperpigmentation

## PIMPLED ASS

P **P**BC
I **I**ron overload[1]
M **M**alignancy[2]
P **P**orphyria cutanea tarda
L **L**iver disease
E **E**ndocrine: 'ACTH'[3]
D **D**rugs: 'BBC 5'[4]

A **A**rsenic
S **S**cleroderma
S **S**prue + other malabsorption states

---

**notes**

1 Especially haemochromatosis (= 'bronze diabetes')
2 Melanoma, malignancy per se and paraneoplastic syndromes (eg ectopic ACTH*)
3 'ACTH':  **A**ddison's
  **C**ushing's
  **T**umours
  **H**yperparathyroidism
  (also ectopic ACTH* + Nelson's syndrome)
4 'BBC 5':  **B**usulphan
  **B**leomycin
  **C**hloroquine
  **5**-Fluorouracil
  (Other: amiodarone/thiazides)

---

# Malignant melanoma

## ABCDE

A **A**symmetry
B **B**order irregularity
C **C**olour variation
D **D**iameter >7 mm (>6 mm in USA guidelines)
E **E**levated above skin

Also bleeding and mild itch

Malar rash

 **SMILER**

S **S**erotonin (carcinoid syndrome)
M **M**itral stenosis (+ other causes of RVH)
I **I**mpetigo: skin infection secondary to *Staphylococcus aureus* or *Streptococcus pyogenes*
L **L**upus: including lupus pernio[1] and vulgaris[2] (spares nasolabial fold)
E **E**rysipelas: skin infection secondary to *Staphylococcus pyogenes* or *Streptococcus pyogenes*
R **R**osacea (acne)

> **notes**
> 1  Lupus pernio: hard and red – caused by sarcoid
> 2  Lupus vulgaris: soft and brown – caused by cutaneous TB

 Pseudoxanthoma elasticum

 **CHICKS**

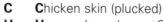

C **C**hicken skin (plucked)
H **H**aemorrhage (upper GI) is associated
I **I**ndigo (blue) sclerae: also can cause angioid streaks
C **C**oronary artery disease
K **K**laudication (in calves, ie PVD)
S **S**queaky valves: MR/AR/aortic dissection

The skin has a 'plucked chicken' appearance

 Acanthosis nigricans

 **PODGE**

P **P**olycystic ovary syndrome
O **O**besity (per se – hence mnemonic!)
D **D**iabetes mellitus
G **G**astric (especially adeno) and other cancers (lymphoma)
E **E**ndocrine (other): Cushing's, acromegaly

> **notes**
>
> Features: increased pigment (brown/black), velvety/soft and warty
>
> Common places: axillae, back of neck and all body folds

# Pyoderma gangrenosum

## Necrotic ULCeR

**Necrotic**   **N**o cause found in 50% (therefore are 'idiopathic')

**U**   **U**C/Crohn's[1]
**L**   **L**eukaemias (including PRV[2])/**L**ymphomas
**C**   **C**irrhosis[3]
**R**   **R**heumatoid arthritis[4]

*Causes ulcers[5] with non-infective necrotic centre*

> **notes**
>
> 1 Can even *precede* the onset of inflammatory bowel disease!
> 2 Multiple myeloma/IgA monoclonal gammopathy
> 3 For example chronic active hepatitis, primary biliary cirrhosis and sclerosing cholangitis
> 4 And rarely other forms of arthritis, especially spondyloarthropathies such as ankylosing spondylitis
> 5 Ulcers occur most commonly on lower limbs (especially shins) and face, but can occur almost anywhere. Characteristic features are ragged purplish overhanging edge (they look like a flattish purple volcano with red lava inside!). Lesions start as a sterile pustule which breaks down and spreads out
>    - Differential diagnosis: infective (exclude with cultures – before treatment!) and vasculitic causes
>    - Diagnosis: biopsy – neutrophil infiltration with haemorrhage and necrosis of epidermis
>    - Treatment: mild ('indolent') cases – topical steroids, intralesional injections of steroids (±minocycline)
>    - Severe (rapidly progressive or painful) cases – high-dose oral steroids (±azathioprine)

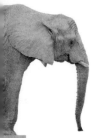

# 10. Neurology

art 1

## Absent ankle jerks and upgoing plantars

### 5Ss

S **S**ubacute combined degeneration of the cord
S **S**yphilis
S **S**pondylosis[1]
S **S**tephen Hawking (ie motor neurone disease[2])
S **S**eparate diseases affecting UMN and LMN[3]

> **notes**
>
> Friedreich's ataxia is the only other cause that doesn't fit into this list
>
> 1 If involves cervical and lumbar regions
> 2 Especially if amyotrophic lateral sclerosis variant
> 3 Simultaneous, common but unrelated diseases, such as a cord lesion (UMN) and diabetic peripheral neuropathy (LMN)

art 1

## Peripheral neuropathy

### ABCDEFGHIIII

A **A**lcohol/**A**rthritis (rheumatoid)/**A**myloid/**A**cromegaly/**A**IP/**A**NA[1]
B **B**$_{12}$* (and folate*) deficiency[2]
C **C**arcinoma*[3]/**C**RF* (+ dialysis per se)
D **D**iabetes*†[4]
E **E**nvironmental toxins: arsenic or lead[5]
F **F**amilial: HSMN[6], Refsum's
G **G**uillain–Barré†[7]

**H** **H**epatic failure
**I** **I**atrogenic: drugs[8]
**I**nfection: TB, Lyme/diphtheria/*Campylobacter*, tetanus/botulism
HIV/EBV/CMV
**I**mmunisations (and foreign serums per se)
**I**diopathic (20% of all cases!!!)

---

**notes**

1 Sjögren's: Ro/La +ve
2 Also ↓ $B_1$ and ↓ or ↑ $B_6$
3 Including myeloma and paraneoplastic (especially if anti-Hu antibodies)
4 Rarely also caused by low glucose (via insulinomas)
5 Wrist + ankle drop common
6 HSMN = hereditary sensorimotor neuropathy (old name = Charcot–Marie–Tooth); there are 4 types:
 ● I:† 'classical type': PMA, sensory ataxia, familial, 1st decade, pes cavus, scoliosis common
 ● II:* milder, presents later (2nd decade), pes cavus rare
 ● III: slow progression, large (thickened) nerves are distinctive feature
 ● IV: rare!
7 Acute inflammatory demyelinating polyradiculopathy (AIDP). Chronic form exists (CIDP), which is a relatively common cause of peripheral neuropathy; is said to occur if weakness continues to develop for more than 4 weeks and tends to run relapsing/remitting course (treat with iv immunoglobulins)
8 CAMP VAN: **C**iclosporin, **A**miodarone, **M**etronidazole, **P**henytoin, **V**incristine*/Cisplatin, **A**mitriptyline, **N**itrofurantoin/Chloramphenicol

*Axonal (EMG: amplitude loss)
†Demyelinating (EMG: conduction velocity loss)

---

**Part 1** Chorea

### WRITHES ABOUT A LOT

**W** **W**ilson's
**R** **R**heumatic fever (= Sydenham's chorea)
**I** **I**atrogenic*[1]
**T** **T**hyrotoxicosis and other endocrine[2]
**H** **H**untingdon's
**E** **E**ncephalitis[3]
**S** **S**LE/**S**enile/**S**trokes/**S**ubdurals

| | |
|---|---|
| **A** | **A**lcohol (intoxication or withdrawal) |
| **B** | **B**enign hereditary*[4]/**B**ilirubin (kernicterus) |
| **O** | **O**estrogens* (Pregnancy or OCP[1]) |
| **U** | **U**lcers (Behçet's) and other autoimmunes[5] |
| **T** | **T**umour/**T**ricyclic antidepressants |

*Commonest causes: oestrogens are rarest of these 3

Rarer causes:

| | |
|---|---|
| **A** | **A**canthocytosis (= **A**betalipoproteinaemia)[6] |
| **L** | **L**esch–Nyhan |
| **O** | **O**xygen deficiency – anoxic damage/cerebral palsy |
| **T** | **T**oxic : CO, manganese, mercury, thallium, toluene |

**notes**

1  L-Dopa, selegiline, antipsychotics, bromocriptine, tricyclic antidepressants, metoclopramide, prochlorperazine and OCP
2  Other endocrine causes: ↓PTH, ↓ or ↑ $Na^+$, ↓ or ↑ glucose
3  Including CJD and encephalitis lethargica
4  aka Congenital juvenile hereditary
5  Other autoimmunes: sarcoid, multiple sclerosis, polyarteritis nodosum, Henoch–Schönlein purpura
6  Also known as Bassen–Kornzweig disease: see p. 92

---

**art 1** Dystrophia myotonica

---

**ACES**

### BALD AT FRONT

| | |
|---|---|
| **B** | **B**ald at front[1]/**B**ilateral ptosis[1] |
| **A** | **A**trophy[1] and weakness/'**A**fter potentials' seen on EMG |
| **L** | **L**et go of my hand![2] |
| **D** | **D**ominant (autosomal)[3]/**D**eep tendon reflexes depressed |
| | |
| **A** | **A**nticipation[3]/**A**rrhythmias[4] |
| **T** | **T**hyroid (and diabetes) |
| | |
| **F** | **F**rontal signs[5] |
| **R** | **R**educed IQ (mild) |
| **O** | **O**cular **O**pacity (= cataracts*!) |
| **N** | **N**ot able to swallow (dysphagia†) |
| **T** | **T**esticular atrophy[6] |

1  Frontal alopecia and bilateral ptosis are most prominent features on inspection. Combined with an expressionless face and muscle wasting (atrophy) of head and neck (especially temporalis, masseters and sternocleidomastoid) they cause the classic 'myotonic facies'

2  Prolonged grip (myotonia) – unable to relax after muscle contraction, eg shaking hand

3  Anticipation: defect is a triplet repeat (CTG on chromosome 19) that expands through generations to reach a 'clinical threshold': often the only feature in older generations is cataracts* before the full phenotype develops (after XX). *Older generations 'anticipate' the later disease!*

4  Including complete heart block – also cardiomyopathy

5  Disinhibited/behavioural problems, ↓ executive function and ↑ primitive reflexes (blink, grasp, palmo-mental, pout, snout)

6  Testicular atrophy ⇒ ↓testosterone ⇒ infertility in middle age and gynaecomastia

Weakness normally first affects hands and feet (causing foot drop) first. Limbs and bulbar† muscles are involved in advanced cases

### Percussion myotonia

● Tap firmly on thenar eminence can use index finger but tendon hammer best. Cautious taps may not illicit this sign; thenar eminence is not tender and you can afford to initially tap hard without hurting patient!

● Same sign can be elicited on the tongue using a tongue depressor

### Treatment

● Quinine, phenytoin, procainamide can help with myotonia but not progression of disease/weakness

---

**Part 1** Mononeuritis multiplex

### DISTAL PATCHeS

| | |
|---|---|
| **D** | **D**iabetes mellitus |
| **I** | **I**mmunisations[1]/**I**njury[2] |
| **S** | **S**LE/**S**jögren's |
| **T** | **T**umour[3] |
| **A** | **A**rthritis (rheumatoid) |
| **L** | **L**yme disease/**L**eprosy |

**P** **P**olyarteritis nodosum
**A** **A**myloid/**A**cromegaly
**T** **T**omaculous[4]/**T** cell depletion (HIV)
**C** **C**hurg–Strauss + Wegener's
**H** **H**erpes zoster
**S** **S**arcoid

*Patch(e)s of neuropathy are seen distally!*

> **notes**
> 1 And other foreign serums
> 2 Radiotherapy or thermal/electrical injury
> 3 Carcinomatosis, malignant nerve tumours, paraproteinaemias
> 4 Genetic syndrome where **T**rivial **T**rauma (such as sleeping on a nerve)
>    causes mononeuropathies which generally resolve, but can progress to
>    general motor and sensory damage

## Predominantly motor neuropathy

### GP PLOD

**G** **G**uillain–Barré[1]
**P** **P**orphyria (acute intermittent)

**P** **P**eroneal muscular atrophy[2]
**L** **L**ead poisoning: see p. 119
**O** **O**rganophosphates
**D** **D**apsone/**D**M (diabetic amyotrophy)/**D**iphtheria

> **notes**
> 1 Acute inflammatory demyelinating polyneuropathy
> 2 = Hereditary sensorimotor neuropathy = Charcot–Marie–Tooth

## Thickened nerves

### HARD Lines

| | |
|---|---|
| **H** | **H**SMN[1]/**H**ypertrophic neuropathy[2] |
| **A** | **A**myloid/**A**cromegaly/**A**IDS |
| **R** | **R**efsum's |
| **D** | **D**iabetes/**D**emyelinating polyradiculopathy[3] |

**Lines** **L**eprosy

> Sarcoid is another rare cause
>
> Best places to see or feel these are: head of fibula (common peroneal), elbow (ulnar) or wrist (radial)
>
> 1 HSMN = Hereditary sensorimotor neuropathy: ***type I (and rarely III) only***
> 2 Rare autosomal dominant condition
> 3 Acute (Guillain–Barré) or chronic (CIDP)

## Median nerve hand muscles

| | |
|---|---|
| **L** | **L**ateral 2 lumbricals |
| **O** | **O**pponens pollicis |
| **A** | **Ab**ductor pollicis brevis[1] |
| **F** | **F**lexor pollicis brevis |

> Median nerve is formed from medial and lateral cords of brachial plexus (roots C6/7/8 and T1)
>
> Also supplies:
>
> - All muscles on front of the forearm *except* flexor carpi ulnaris and flexor digitorum profundus (inner/ulnar half of)
> - Sensation from lateral (radial) 3½ fingers
>
> 1 This is the best muscle to test – with their palm facing up ask patient to point thumbs to the sky and resist your pushing them down with your thumbs

# Ulnar nerve hand muscles

## MAFIA

**M** Medial lumbricals
**A** Adductor pollicis (transverse and oblique heads of)
**F** Flexor pollicis brevis (inner head of)
**I** Interossei[1]
**A** Abductor digiti minimi + hypothenar eminence

1 First dorsal interosseous can be supplied by the median nerve

Formed from medial cord of brachial plexus (roots are C7/8)

Also supplies:

- Muscles in forearm: flexor carpi ulnaris and flexor digitorum profundus (inner/ulnar half of)
- Sensation from medial (ulnar) 1½ fingers

---

# (Proximal) myopathy

## Polly's Perilous Thighs Could Crush Al's Muscular Midriff Ostentatiously

| | |
|---|---|
| **Polly's** | **Poly**myositis/dermatomyositis[1] |
| **Perilous** | **Peri**odic paralysis |
| **Thighs** | **Th**yroid/DM (including amyotrophy that is asymmetrical) |
| **Could** | **Co**rticosteroids[2] (exogenous) |
| **Crush** | **Cush**ing's syndrome (any cause of) |
| **Al's** | **Al**cohol |
| **Muscular** | **Muscular** dystrophy |
| **Midriff** | **M**yasthenia gravis |
| **Ostentatiously** | **Oste**omalacia[3] |

**notes**

NB *Not* caused by polymyalgia rheumatica; causes pain and stiffness *but not weakness*!

1. Look for heliotrope rash ('violaceous' rash around eyes) and Gottron's papules (scaly erythematous lesions) over dorsal aspect of hands (especially knuckles)
2. Other drugs include statins/fibrates, antimalarials (chloroquine, hydroxychloroquine), penicillamine, retrovirals. Rarely cytotoxics, antibiotics, narcotics and ACE inhibitors
3. Look for bone pain, skeletal deformity and waddling gait

**Part 1** Ptosis (causes of)

**PACES**

## MITCH

| | |
|---|---|
| **M** | **M**yasthenia gravis |
| **I** | **I**diopathic |
| **T** | **T**hird nerve palsy |
| **C** | **C**ongenital |
| **H** | **H**orner's* |

**notes**

Bilateral causes: above plus mitochondrial dystrophy, myotonic dystrophy, oculopharyngeal dystrophy, ocular myopathy, syphilis, botulism, migraine or cluster headaches (especially if paroxysmal) or Horner's (*more likely to be bilateral if due to a syrinx see p. 56)

**Part 1** Internuclear ophthalmoplegia

**PACES**

| A**B**ducting eye | **B**eats |
|---|---|
| A**D**ducting eye | **D**elayed |

*The ab*ducting eye ***beats*** *and therefore exhibits nystagmus, and the ad*ducting eye shows ***delayed*** *movement and is therefore slower in moving than the abducting eye*

notes

Is caused by damage to the medial longitudinal fasciculus (MLF), the connection between the nuclei of the third and fourth cranial nerves which coordinates the two nerves in eye movements

An internuclear ophthalmoplegia (INO) is elicited by saccadic (as opposed to pursuit) eye movements – ask the patient to switch instantly, whilst keeping the head stationary, from looking at your face (directly in front of the patient) to an outstretched hand (at the extreme of vision on either side)

## Cerebellar syndrome (causes)

### CINNAMON

| | |
|---|---|
| C | **C**VA |
| I | **I**nherited*: especially Friedrich's and SCAs[1] |
| N | **N**eoplasms: 1° (rarely 2°) |
| N | **N**eoplasms: paraneoplastic*[2] |
| A | **A**nticonvulsants* (especially phenytoin) |
| M | **M**ultiple sclerosis |
| O | **O**titis media (if severe and causes abscess) |
| N | **N**utritional deficiency*[3] |

notes

*Tend to be bilateral and symmetrical. The others can be, but less commonly

1 Spinocerebellar ataxias (many types exist)
2 Especially secondary to lung and breast antineuronal antibodies: easy to forget and not rare so deserves the second mention of neoplasms!
3 Alcohol, pellagra, amoebiasis, protracted vomiting

## Cerebellar signs

### DANISH

| | |
|---|---|
| D | **D**ysdiadokokinesis/**D**ysmetria[1] |
| A | **A**taxia of gait[2] (and trunk[3]) |
| N | **N**ystagmus[4] |
| I | **I**ntention tremor[5] |
| S | **S**lurred **S**peech[6] |
| H | **H**ypotonia[7] (**H**yporeflexia[8]) |

1 Dysmetria = past pointing. Also look for 'rebound': overshooting up (or down) of hands past horizontal when pushed down (or up) with eyes closed
2 Broad based and unsteady with irregular step length
3 If lesion to cerebellar vermis (hemispheric lesions cause gait ataxia)
4 Is horizontal, towards side of lesion and classically 'coarse' (big jumps)
5 Also look for titubation ('nodding head' tremor)
6 'Cerebellar dysarthria'; also described as **S**tuttering, **S**taccato or **S**canning
7 Hypotonia is secondary to loss of facilitatory influence of spinal motor neurones
8 Less common and often described as 'pendular' reflexes

**Examination routine**

- There are many ways of looking for all these features – perhaps the slickest way is to start at the top of the body and work down: mouth (speech), eyes (nystagmus), hands (dysdiadochokinesis, finger-nose, rebound), legs (gait).
- Arms (hypotonia, hyporeflexia) are probably best left as a 'To complete my examination I'd like to' add-on, as are 'softer signs' and have many other causes.
- Whatever routine you settle on it is best to start with speech as this gives you time to fully observe the patient (and bedside) whilst asking a few friendly (rapport and point gaining) questions before honing in on more specific speech questions.
- Commenting on symmetry will score more points and allow a more focused differential diagnosis (see CINNAMON above)

 Friedreich's ataxia

 **Cerebellar** signs[1]

## PADUNCLES

| | |
|---|---|
| **P** | **P**es cavus[2]/**P**ale discs (optic atrophy) |
| **A** | **A**utosomal recessive[3] |
| **D** | **D**iabetes (in 10%; more have ↓ glucose tolerance) |
| **U** | **U**pper motor neurone signs in limbs[4] |
| **N** | **N**europathy (peripheral sensory)[5] |
| **C** | **C**ardiomyopathy[6] |
| **L** | **L**oss of posterior columns[7], hearing and sphincter function |
| **E** | **E**xcellent IQ (ie normal; rarely mild cognitive impairment) |
| **S** | **S**coliosis (mostly as kyphoscoliosis) |

*Cerebellar signs predominate (hence the name ataxia!); note
deliberate misspelling of peduncles (the part of the cerebellum
that attaches to the brainstem)*

**notes**

1 See previous mnemonic. Especially progressive gait ataxia (before 30
years old) and intention tremor then dysarthria later
2 Occurs in 50%. Other foot deformities occur such as high arched feet (not
reaching level of pes cavus), foot inversion and hammer toes
3 Chromosome 9 trinucleotide (GAA) repeat expansion: males and females
equally affected
4 Upgoing plantars*, weakness (and loss of abdominal reflexes)
5 Loss of reflexes (ankles* then knees) and distal wasting
6 Hypertrophic cardiomyopathy in 50%. Causes heart failure and
arrhythmias
7 Joint position sense + vibration distally

*Friedreich's is therefore a cause of absent ankle jerks and upgoing plantars
(see p. 69)

# Bilateral lower motor neurone VII lesion

## BILAT Seven

| | |
|---|---|
| B | **B**ell's palsy[1] (HSV/HZV) |
| I | **I**nflammatory myositis[2] |
| L | **L**yme |
| A | **A**IDP[3]/**A**LS[4] |
| T | **T**etanus (cephalitic) |
| **Seven** | **S**arcoid |

> **notes**
>
> Unilateral causes:
>
> - LMN – above, plus: tumour (especially cerebellopontine angle + parotid), trauma, mononeuritis multiplex, pontine lesions (multiple sclerosis/CVA), middle ear disease (deafness), polio, HIV, TB, diabetes mellitus, pregnancy
> - UMN – CVA, tumour
>
> 1 Causes unilateral lesions much more commonly!
> 2 Also muscular dystrophy
> 3 Acute inflammatory demyelinating polyneuropathy (= Guillain–Barré syndrome)
> 4 Amyotrophic lateral sclerosis (= type of motor neurone disease)

**Part 1** Demyelinating diseases

**PACES** **Pissed AS A GNAT**

| | |
|---|---|
| **Pissed** | Alcohol: Wernicke's (+ Korsakoff's) encephalopathies |
| **A** | **A**cute haemorrhagic leukoencephalopathy/**A**IDS[1] |
| **S** | **S**chindler's* |
| **A** | **A**cute disseminated encephalomyelitis |
| **G** | **G**aucher's* |
| **N** | **N**iemann–Pick*/**N**euromyelitis optica |
| **A** | **A**dreno (or metachromatic) Leukodystrophy* |
| **T** | **T**ay–Sachs*/**T**ropical spastic paraparesis[2] |

> **notes**
>
> The most common (and too obvious to need learning) cause is, of course, multiple sclerosis!
>
> Rarer causes are: central pontine demyelination, phenylketonuria, carbon monoxide/mercury poisoning, hypoxia, $B_{12}$ deficiency (linked to Wernicke's/Korsakoff's above), Binswanger's (vascular), Krabbe's*, Alexander's
>
> Krabbes*/Alexanders
>
> 1 Also remember the leukoencephalopathy that is an AIDS-defining illness: progressive multifocal leukoencephalopathy
> 2 Similar disease to multiple sclerosis caused by HTLV-1 virus
>
> *Lipid storage diseases

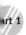

# Winging of the scapula

## SALT BAR 567

**S** **S**erratus muscle affected
**A** **A**nterior muscle affected
**L** **L**ong nerve supplying it
**T** **T**horacic nerve supplying it

of

**B** **B**ell long thoracic nerve of Bell is other name
**A** **A**nterior
**R** **R**ami

of

**567** **C** 5/6/7

> Resistance when outstretched arms are pushed forward causes inner portion of the scapula to 'wing out' or be displaced away from the chest wall. Also causes inability to raise the arm overhead
>
> Long thoracic nerve is damaged by injury (eg carrying heavy weights on the shoulder), diabetes, neuralgic amyotrophy or systemic disorders
>
> Need to exclude muscular dystrophy before diagnosis!

# CT brain ring enhancing lesions

## SNATCH

**S** **S**mall abscesses
**N** **N**eoplasms[1]
**A** **A**spergilloma
**T** **T**B/**T**oxoplasmosis/**T**hrombosed arteriovenous malformations
**C** **C**ysticercosis[2]
**H** **H**ydatid disease[3]/**H**amartoma (resolving)

> Seen when contrast given and accumulates around a structure
>
> 1 Primaries, metastases and CNS lymphomas (especially in AIDS)
> 2 Name for when *Taenia solium* (pork tapeworm) larvae enter tissues
> 3 *Echinococcus* tapeworms

**Part 1** Wilson's

 **Part 2** **BRAIN**

**B** **B**asal ganglia involvement[1]
**R** **R**enal tubular acidosis: type II (proximal) and $HCO_3^-$ loss
**A** **A**cute haemolysis[2]/**A**menorrhoea
**I** **I**ris: KF (Kayser–Fleischer) rings[3]
**N** **N**europsychiatric features[4]

*And liver (cirrhosis with copper deposition) are organs affected most!*

---

**notes**

1 Basal ganglia involvement causing movement disorders: especially dystonia but also tremor, postural abnormalities and rarely chorea. Cerebellar features (dysarthria, ↓ coordination/gait) can also occur
2 Rare in reality but common in MRCP!
3 Brown/green deposits in limbus of cornea; most easily seen in blue iris – slit lamp needed to exclude. Are said to always be present if there is neurological impairment. Can also be seen in other disorders causing prolonged cholestasis, such as PBC
4 Especially psychosis and personality change; can be presenting feature!

**Diagnosis**

- KF rings + serum caeruloplasmin <20 mg/l (or <200 mg/l + liver biopsy with >250 μg/g of copper)
- To fully exclude diagnosis, liver biopsy needed; causes ↑Cu + fatty changes (mimics EtOH disease and Cu also seen deposited in PBC)

---

 **Part 1** Berry aneurysm associations

**TINS OF PEACH**

**T** **T**uberose sclerosis
**I** **I**nfective endocarditis
**N** **N**eurofibromatosis (type I)
**S** **S**ickle/**S**LE

**O** **O**ther collagen type III disorders
**F** **F**ibromuscular dysplasia

**P**   **P**seudoxanthoma elasticum
**E**   **E**hlers–Danlos (and Marfan's)
**A**   **A**dult polycystic kidney disease/AVMs/ $\alpha_1$ antitrypsin
**C**   **C**oarctation
**H**   **H**ereditary haemorrhagic telangiectasia[1]

*'PEACH' covers the most common causes*

> **notes**
>
> Aka 'Saccular' or congenital aneurysms: most are asymptomatic but are common (5% of the population, of which one-third have multiple) and cause 80% of subarachnoid haemorrhages
>
> 1  = Osler–Weber–Rendu syndrome

## Increased CSF protein but normal cells

**GLASS**

**G**   **G**uillain–Barré
**L**   **L**ead poisoning
**A**   **A**coustic neuroma
**S**   **S**ubacute sclerosing panaencephalitis[1]
**S**   **S**pinal cord tumour[2]/meningitis[2]

> **notes**
>
> 1  Persistence of measles antigen in CNS: causes progressive pyramidal signs, myoclonic jerks, convulsions, cognitive/behavioural change and eventually death
> 2  Can also cause xanthochromia. When this is combined with normal cells and ↑ protein = Froin's syndrome

## Guillain–Barré syndrome infective causes

### CMV

C *Campylobacter jejuni*[1]
M *Mycoplasma pneumoniae*
V Viruses (other):

- Coxsackie virus
- Hepatitis/HIV
- Influenza/Infectious mononucleosis
- Measles
- Paramyxovirus (mumps)

*CMV virus is the most common cause!*

---

**notes**

### Rarer causes

- Immunisations, surgery, trauma, autoimmune disorders (accounts for 2.5% of cases, eg SLE and RA) and very rarely malignancy

### Features

- Autonomic: heart (hypertension, arrhythmias), GI (pain), bladder atony
- Pain: severe lumbar/interscapular pain
- Paraesthesia (sensory signs rare!)

### Miller fisher variant

- External ophthalmoplegia, ataxia, areflexia

1 Other GI infections can cause it, especially *Salmonella*

---

## Horner's syndrome

### PAMELA

P Ptosis
A Anhidrosis[1]
M Miosis: small pupil[2]
E Enophthalmos: sunken eye[3]
L Loss of ciliospinal reflex[4]
A Any scars[5]? Clues to Aetiology[6]

**PAM** describes the standard triad (note anhidrosis not always present[1]) and **ELA** are extra things you can talk about/try to demonstrate if you want to show off!

*This mnemonic sticks in the mind if you think envisage a **Horny** (Horner's) **PAMELA** Anderson!*

Ptosis and/or miosis should alert you to this condition in PACES exam; it is easy to miss when nervous so take your time to compare for asymmetry. Can come up in CNS, eyes or as part of respiratory (Pancoast's) stations

1 Occurs if lesion is proximal to the superior cervical ganglion, ie 'central'. Can be differentiated from 'proximal' causes with cocaine and adrenaline drops. If central cocaine dilates both pupils and adrenaline has no effect on either eye. If peripheral cocaine dilates normal eye but not affected one and adrenaline does the opposite

2 With preservation of light and accommodation reflex. Remember Argyll Robertson (syphilitic) pupils accommodate normally but lose light reflex

3 NB This isn't *true* enophthalmos

4 Aka papillary-skin reflex: pupil dilation if pin scratched on same side of the neck: unreliable and painful!

5 Remember to look for any scars (and expose clavicle if not visible) for clues of cause

6 Causes: start at origin of sympathetic nucleus in brainstem (*CVA, Wallenberg's, MS, tumour, syringobulbia*), follow path down cord (syringomyelia, trauma) and out at C8, T1, T2 (*any lesions at this level*) having synapsed with pre-ganglionic neurones to T1 ganglion (*Pancoast's tumour*) and up sympathetic chain (*trauma/surgery/lymph nodes*) to superior cervical ganglion (where synapses with postganglionic fibres) which travel up neck (*trauma, surgery*) to carotid plexus (*aneurysm, dissection, occlusion or carotid body tumour*) and then into orbit where joins ciliary ganglion and exits as long and short ciliary nerves to dilator pupillae (*orbital tumour/trauma*). Note parasympathetic (constricting) supply also enters ciliary ganglion as part of occulomotor nerve (CnIII)

NB Cause can be *congenital*, in which case one would expect to see heterochromia (affected eye remains blue when normal eye turns brown under control of sympathetic nervous system during development), or due to *migraine or cluster headaches* if paroxysmal presentation

Parkinson's disease

## ART FILMS

A    **A**kinesia[*1]
R    **R**igidity[*2]
T    **T**remor[*3]

F    **F**rontal reflexes[4]/**F**acies: blank or expressionless
I    **I**nvoluntary movements (dyskinesias[5])
L    **L**oss of balance: ↓postural reflexes[6]
M    **M**icrographia[7]
S    **S**huffling gait[8]

---

**notes**

\*Are the 3 core features (NB belong to 'akinetic–rigid syndromes').
Asymmetry favours idiopathic Parkinson's over drug-induced.

### Parkinson's plus syndromes

- Look for supranuclear palsy (eyes look up further via reflexes when head tilted forwards than they can voluntarily) or progressive supranuclear palsy (aka Steele–Richardson) and ask for evidence of autonomic dysfunction (postural hypotension, urinary symptoms and impotence) in multi system atrophy (aka Shy–Drager)

1 Akinesia/bradykinesia: best seen in speed of sequential movement of thumb to all finger tips
2 Remember 'lead pipe' is the classic description; becomes 'cogwheeling' if tremor is superimposed on this
3 Tremor at 20 Hz (favourite banal question of examiners!), classically with 'pill rolling' action. Distraction (eg counting backwards) and resting forearms on arms of chair can help bring out subtle cases
4 Frontal reflexes: glabellar tap (blink), pout, root (suckling), grasp and palmo-mental
5 Especially chorea and dystonias related to L-dopa, mostly at peak dose when 'on'
6 Good in assessing function (risk of falls) as are doing up buttons or writing
7 Drawing a spiral or writing name
8 Also "festinant", ↓ armswing, slow starting and poor turning

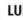

# Mitochondrial diseases

## LUMP

**L** **L**imb girdle myopathy/**L**eber's (see p. 89)/**L**eigh disease[1]
**U** **U**sher's syndrome[2]
**M** **M**ELLAS[3]/**M**ERRF[4]
**P** **P**rogressive external ophthalmoplegia[5]

---

Mitochondrial diseases have a unique pattern of inheritance – can only come from mother! They affect organs highly dependent on oxidative metabolism: muscles (most commonly causing myopathy but can also affect heart and GI tract) and brain (causing a wide spectrum of neurological disorders). Often cause distinctive signs such as retinitis pigmentosa – see p. 91

1 Leigh disease: subacute necrotising encephalomyopathy, retinitis pigmentosa, weakness, ataxia and cognitive impairment
2 Usher's syndrome: autosomal recessive disease characterised by sensorineural deafness (non-progressive)
3 MELLAS: **M**itochondrial **E**ncephalopathy, **L**actic **A**cidosis and **S**troke-like episodes (myopathy also seen)
4 MERRF: **M**yoclonic **E**pilepsy with **R**ed **R**agged **F**ibres (histological appearance of muscle biopsy)
5 Kearns–Sayre syndrome is the extreme form of this: triad of progressive external ophthalmoplegia, heart block and retinitis pigmentosa

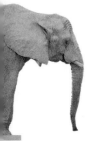

# 11. Ophthalmology

## Optic atrophy

### DISC PALLOR

| | |
|---|---|
| **D** | **D**emyelination (especially MS) |
| **I** | **I**ntraocular pressure (ie glaucoma!) |
| **S** | **S**yphilis (*Tabes*)/**S**enile macular degeneration |
| **C** | **C**ompression of optic nerve[1] |
| **P** | **P**apilloedema (prolonged)/**P**aget's |
| **A** | **A**cute ischaemic optic neuritis/**A**rteritis (temporal) |
| **L** | **L**eber's + other hereditary causes[2] |
| **L** | **L**ead and other poisoning[3] |
| **O** | **O**cclusion of retinal artery |
| **R** | **R**etinitis pigmentosa: see p. 91 |

*Pale (white) discs are seen on fundoscopy!*

---

1 Tumour: pituitary meningioma thyroid , Cn II, carotid aneurysm
2 Friedreich's (see p. 78) and DIDMOAD (diabetes insipidus and mellitus +
  optic atrophy)
3 Arsenic, methanol, tobacco, quinine, ethambutol, $B_{12}$ deficiency

Part 1 Papilloedema

## DISC SWELLING

| D | **D**estruction of retinal vein or artery (occlusion/thromboembolism) |
|---|---|
| I | **I**ntracranial pressure[1] |
| S | **S**evere hypertension (grade IV) |
| C | $CO_2$ retention/**C**hronic optic neuritis[2] |
| | |
| S | **S**teroids[3]/**S**VC obstruction/**S**yphilis/**S**ubhyaloid haemorrhage |
| W | **W**aldenstrom's macroglobulinaemia |
| E | **E**ncephalitis/meningitis |
| L | **L**ead and other poisons (arsenic, MetOH) |
| L | **L**ow Hb (anaemia) |
| I | **I**ncreased Hb (ie PRV) and also other haematological disorders[4] |
| N | **N**eoplasms outside of brain[5] |
| G | **G**uillain–Barré, **G**rave's disease (or any thyroid eye disease) or hypoparathyroidism |

*Swollen discs (with blurred edges) are seen on fundoscopy!*

---

1 Tumour, benign intracranial hypertension, ↑vitamin A, trauma, anoxia, cavernous sinus thrombosis, SAH, aqueduct stenosis
2 Aka 'papillitis': isolated lesion, MS, TB, syphilis, sarcoid
3 Especially in children after withdrawal from steroids
4 DIC, thrombotic thrombocytopenic purpura, sickle
5 Leukaemia, spinal cord tumours* or any spinal block*

*Causes of ↑ CSF protein

---

Scotoma

## SCOTOMA

| S | **S**enile macular degeneration |
|---|---|
| C | **C**ompression of nerve |
| O | **O**ptic neuritis |
| T | **T**oxins |
| O | **O**lfactory groove meningioma |
| M | **M**alignancy (optic nerve glioma) |
| A | **A**lcohol (thiamine deficiency) |

# Retinal vein thrombosis

## DGH

**D** **D**iabetes mellitus
**G** **G**laucoma
**H** **H**ypertension/**H**yperviscosity syndromes*

*Retinal vein thrombosis is relatively common – therefore seen in DGHs!*

> *For example, polycythaemia rubra vera, multiple myeloma, Waldenstrom's macroglobulinemia
>
> ● It can be confused with gross papilloedema (both cause gross 'splatting' of disc!): easiest distinguishing feature is retional vein thrombosis that haemorrhages go out to the extremes of the retina

# Retinitis pigmentosa

## BLACK Network Under Retina

**B** **B**assen-Kornzweig syndrome[1]/**B**atten's syndrome[2]
**L** **L**aurence–Moon–Biedl–Bardet syndrome[3]
**A** **A**utosomal dominant (sporadic) cases – generally more benign
**C** **C**ockayne syndrome*/**C**hronic external ophthalmoplegia*
**K** **K**earns–Sayre syndrome*

**Network** **N**ARP syndrome* (**N**europathic **A**taxia and **R**etinitis **P**igmentosa)

**Under** **U**sher's syndrome*

**Retina** **R**efsum's syndrome[4]

*Black pigment 'network' is seen under retina!*

notes

The appearance is described as 'bone-like' spicules; these occur in Bruch's membrane and start peripherally (spreading in) and are easily remembered once seen, but it is easy to not look far enough out. The optic disc is also pale and therefore not checking peripherally can lead to a mistaken diagnosis of optic atrophy[†]

The major functional impairment is tunnel vision so always check (or ask to check) visual fields. Also causes 'night blindness' ($\downarrow$ vision at dusk), often before detectable on fundoscopy.

### Differential diagnosis

The above appearance is quite distinctive but if unsure consider the following:

- Racial pigmentation of retina: common and not to be mistaken (aka 'tigroid fundus')
- Disseminated melanoma
- Diabetic retinopathy laser burns
- Secondary retinitis pigmentosa (follows inflammatory retinitis)
- [†]Optic atrophy

1 Bassen–Kornzweig syndrome (= acanthocytosis = abetalipoproteinaemia): autosomal recessive metabolic disorder in which malabsorption and spinocerebellar degeneration predominate. Very low cholesterol and triglycerides seen, as well as 'acanthocytes' (spiky red cells) on blood film; 3 separate 'wet' films needed to exclude. Common in Ashkenazi Jews

2 Batten's syndrome (= lipofuscinosis = amaurotic familial idiocy): autosomal recessive (chromosome 16) lysosomal storage defect. Progressive dementia, seizures, spastic weakness, ataxia and athetosis

3 Laurence–Moon–Biedl–Bardet syndrome: autosomal recessive disorder characterised by obesity/DM, visual loss, squint, cataracts, mental retardation, spastic paraplegia, polydactyly, hypogonadism, dwarfism, renal abnormalities

4 Refsum's disease: autosomal recessive loss of phytanic acid, which breaks down chlorophyll. Causes demyelination resulting in motor and sensory neuropathy, cerebellar ataxia, sensorineural deafness, pupillary abnormalities, anosmia, cardiomyopathy, ichthyosis and optic atrophy. Is also a cause of isolated rise in CSF protein (ie normal cell count!)

*Mitochondrial diseases (see p. 87)

# Angioid streaks

## SLAPPERS

| | |
|---|---|
| **S** | **S**ickle*[1] |
| **L** | **L**ead poisoning |
| **A** | **A**betalipoproteinaemia[2]/**A**cromegaly[3] |
| **P** | **P**aget's*/**P**hacomatoses[4] |
| **P** | **P**seudoxanthoma elasticum* |
| **E** | **E**hlers–Danlos |
| **R** | **R**aised calcium or phosphate |
| **S** | **S**hort people (dwarfism) |

- **NB 50% are idiopathic and not associated with any disease.** Can also be caused by trauma
- Are made by 'cracks' in Bruch's membrane (connective tissue layer under retina): red/grey relatively feint but relatively thick (normally at least twice the width of an artery) lines found near retinal vessels, for which they can often be mistaken

*Most common causes, especially pseudoxanthoma elasticum, therefore look for loose 'chicken skin' (especially neck and axillae) and absent pulses (are arteriopaths)

1  Other haemoglobinopathies can also cause this; thalassaemias, spherocytosis
2  Bassen–Kornzweig syndrome = acanthocytosis: see p. 92
3  And other pituitary/endocrine disorders (rarely diabetes and 'bronze diabetes', ie haemochromatosis)
4  Phacomatoses: tuberous sclerosis, neurofibromatosis, Sturge–Weber

# Roth's spots

## PALE Centre

| | |
|---|---|
| **P** | **P**ernicious anaemia |
| **A** | **A**NCA (Vasculitis) |
| **L** | **L**upus |
| **E** | **E**ndocarditis |
| **Centre** | **C**ollagen vascular disease |

*Red haemorrhagic spots with **pale centre**!*

# Cherry red spots

## SPOT

**S**   **S**phingolipidoses: Gaucher's, Tay–Sachs, Niemann–Pick
**P**   *Plasmodium* infection (eg malaria) – due to quinine treatment
**O**   **O**cclusion of retinal artery*
**T**   **T**raumatic oedema

> More prominent red macula spot (normally slightly red with pale centre – like a skin spot!)
>
> *Surrounding ischaemia makes fovea look relatively red

# Old choroidoretinitis

## 6Ts

**T**   **T**oxoplasmosis
**T**   *Toxocara*
**T**   **T**B (also Sarcoid and Behçet's)
**T**   **T**rauma/surgery (and retinal detachment)
**T**   **T** cell depletion (HIV[1])
**T**   *Tabes* (syphilis)

> Aka 'scarring of retina'
>
> NB Laser burns in treated proliferative diabetic retinopathy can have the same appearance but are smaller, rounder, more widespread and often in peripheries (if done near macular will always be very small and subtle so as not to have disturbed vision)
>
> 1   HIV especially common if has been complicated by CMV infection (initially causes 'cottage cheese and ketchup' appearance) but can scar once treated/resolved

# Blue sclera

## Thin Purple Membrane Covering Over Eyes

| | |
|---|---|
| **Thin**[1] | **T**hyrotoxicosis |
| **Purple** | **P**seudoxanthoma elasticum |
| **Membrane** | **M**arfan's |
| **Covering** | **C**orticosteroids (long-term use) |
| **Over** | **O**steogenesis imperfecta[2] |
| **Eyes** | **E**hlers–Danlos |

> **notes**
>
> 1 Thin reminds you of the cause of blue sclerae; which is of thin slera that allows the blue colour of the underlying epithelium to show through
> 2 Most common cause: mostly seen in type I (and II although this is fatal and therefore not seen in adults)

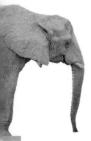

# 12. Psychiatry

## ICD-10 features of depression

### DEPRESSION

| | |
|---|---|
| **D** | **D**epressed mood* |
| **E** | **E**nergy loss* $\Rightarrow$ fatiguability (after slight effort) and $\downarrow$ activity |
| **P** | **P**leasure loss*; interest and enjoyment |
| **R** | **R**etardation (psychomotor); NB rarely agitation can occur instead |
| **E** | **E**ating change: appetite/weight |
| **S** | **S**leep disturbance (early morning waking) |
| **S** | **S**uicidal/self-harm thoughts |
| **I** | **I**nterest/pleasure/enjoyment loss (anhedonia) (**I**'m a failure; loss of confidence/self-esteem) |
| **O** | **O**nly me to blame (guilt/unworthiness) |
| **N** | **N**o concentration or attention |

> **notes**
>
> *'Core' symptoms: 2 of these 3 required for diagnosis
>
> **Mild episode**
>
> - Plus ≥2 of the others *but none present to an intense degree.*
> - Should cause distress and difficulty continuing with ordinary social/work activities, but will probably not cease to function completely
>
> **Moderate**
>
> - Plus ≥3 (preferably 4) of the others, likely to be to a marked degree
> - Usually has considerable difficulty in continuing with social/work activities

> **Severe**
>
> - Plus ≥4 of others, some of which should be of severe intensity
> - Considerable distress/agitation (unless retardation main feature); if so description of symptoms may not be possible and grading may still be justified
> - Low self-esteem or guilt prominent and suicide a distinct danger in particularly severe cases
> - Somatic syndrome almost always present
> - ±Psychotic episode
>
> Symptoms need to be present for 2 weeks (not strictly necessary for severe episode of rapid onset). Are defined ± somatic syndrome: see below

# Somatic (biological) features of depression

## ICD-10

## SOMATIC

| | |
|---|---|
| **S** | **S**leep disturbance; **S**pecifically early morning waking[1] |
| **O** | **O**bjective psychomotor disturbance[2] |
| **M** | **M**orning mood worse (diurnal variation) |
| **A** | **A**ppetite loss/weight loss[3] (count as 1 each!) |
| **T** | **T**empered emotional reactivity[4] |
| **I** | **I**nterest and pleasure loss[5] |
| **C** | **C**elibate; marked loss of libido |

> 1  Defined as ≥2 h before usual time
> 2  Objectivity is important – needs to be remarked on or reported by others. Psychomotor retardation is typical but rarely agitation can occur
> 3  Defined as ≥5% of weight in last month
> 4  To normally pleasurable surroundings or events
> 5  In activities that are usually enjoyable
>
> Usually this syndrome is not regarded as present unless ≥4 of these 8 symptoms are *definitely* present. If there are 2 or 3 which are unusually severe this can suffice

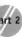

# Mania

## MANIAC

| | |
|---|---|
| **M** | **M**ood increase: elation/euphoria[1] |
| **A** | **A**ctivity/energy increase: mental and physical |
| **N** | **N**o inhibitions/**N**aughty: disinhibited[2] |
| **I** | **I**nsomnia: reduced need for sleep |
| **A** | **A**lways talking[3] |
| **C** | **C**onfidence (optimism) excess[4] |

---

**notes**

1 Can be replaced by irritability, conceit or 'boorishness'
2 Disinhibition: over familiar, overspending, sexual disinhibition
3 'Pressure of speech' and 'flight of ideas'
4 Can progress to 'grandiosity', which can then progress to a 'delusional intensity'

### ICD-10 diagnosis

- Mood change 'should' be accompanied by increased energy and several symptoms, particularly: pressure of speech, sleeplessness (decreased need for), grandiosity and excessive optimism
- Must have episode for ≥1week and must '*disrupt ordinary work and social activities more or less completely*'

NB Hypomania is an intermediate state between normality and mania without delusions, hallucinations or complete disruption of normal activities

Can be psychotic (hallucinations or delusions – often grandiose or religious)

---

# Korsakoff's

## ADICT

| | |
|---|---|
| **A** | **A**mnesia (anterograde[1] especially) |
| **D** | **D**isorientation |
| **I** | **I**nsight loss |
| **C** | **C**onfabulation |
| **T** | **T**hiamine deficiencies[2] |

---

**notes**

1 No new memories since onset
2 Most commonly seen in alcoholics, but also in eating disorders or if chronic vomiting or malnutrition of other cause (rare in the UK)

Narcolepsy

## Part 2

**NARC**

**N** **N**arcolepsy[1] 100%
**A** **A**uditory hallucinations[2] 30%
**R** **R**igid in sleep (= sleep paralysis) 40%
**C** **C**ataplexy[3] 90%

---

This is a classic 'tetrad' – although narcolepsy itself is the only feature required for diagnosis – the others are seen in variable percentages of cases as above

1 Narcolepsy = sudden and irresistable urges to sleep; are refreshing
2 Also see visual hallucinations but less commonly. Can be hypno**go**gic (on **go**ing to sleep) or hypno**po**mpic (on waking from sleep)
3 Sudden loss of muscle tone; often causes collapse and commonly precipitated by emotions (laughter/stress). NB Don't confuse with *catalepsy* (type of catatonia) – the only "lepsy" allowed is the name of the condition itself!

### Associations

- Affective and personality disorders in 50%
- HLA-DR2 (DR15/DQ6) +ve in 99.5%

### Genetics

- Increased risk in first-degree relative (40×)
- Onset aged 10–20: can occur earlier but rare after middle age
- REM onset in first stage of sleep, ↑ stage 1, ↑ number of wakenings

### Treatment

- Stimulants (eg methylphenidate/dexamphetamine) – helps narcolepsy but not cataplexy
- SSRIs and TCAs help cataplexy but not sleep problems

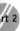

## Anorexia

### Increases = Nucleic Acid bases!

*G and C (guanine and cytosine) pair together and denote the hormonal changes:*
**G** **G**rowth hormone
**C** **C**ortisol (does suppress with dexamethasone)/**C**holesterol

*A and T (adenine and thymine) pair together and denote the GI changes:*
**A** **A**mylase (and even sometimes pancreatitis)
**T** **T**ransaminases: AST and ALT

*Uracil is the base that replaces thymine in RNA:*
**U** **U**rea/Creatine (ie renal failure – can be pre acute or chronic)

### Everything else decreases!

- HR, BP, heart size (also arrhythmias, especially if there are electrolyte abnormalities, and heart failure*); although QTc can increase!
- WCC (although a *relative* lymphocytosis can be seen), Hb (normocytic normochromic 'chronic disease' or microcytic 'Fe deficient')
- K, Ca, $PO_4$, Mg, Zn, glucose, plasma proteins (albumin, etc: explains ankle oedema*)
- Gonadotrophin, oestrogen, testosterone
- $T_3$ and BMR (and temperature)
- Bone density (osteoporosis), GI slowing (↓ gastric emptying and constipation)

## Alzheimer's

### All the As

#### Main (cognitive) features

**A** **A**mnesia – especially "autobiographical"; recent before remote memories
**A** **A**phasia – especially 'nominal' (inability to name things; starts as dysphasia progressing to syntax problems then aphasia
**A** **A**gnosia – difficulty recognising and naming objects, including one's own face

**A**        **A**praxia: problems with complex motor tasks despite the intact basic motor functioning (eg dressing)

**Others**:  **A**ltered personality, **A**nhedonia – depression/mood disturbance

### Investigations

**A**        **A**trophy on MRI: generalised but most significantly in hippocampi

**A**        **A**bnormal EEG: diffuse slowing in early stages, reduced **A**lpha and beta/increased delta and theta later, paroxysmal bifrontal delta waves (more common than in normal aging[1])

### Pathology

**A**        **A**myloid (amyloid AB or B/A4) plaques – extracellular!

**A**        **A**lso neurofibrillary tangles: intracellular

**A**        **A**lso seen in **P**unches:

                boxing induced dementia

                **P**ostencephalitic **P**arkinsonism

                **P**rogressive Supranuclear **P**alsy

**A**        **A**lso Tau/Ubiquitin

### Treatment

**A**        **A**cetylcholinesterase inhibitors, eg donepezil (= **A**ricept), rivastigmine, galantamine

**A**        **A**ntagonists of NMDA (memantine) – note 2× **A** to remember it's an **a**nta**g**onist, not an **a**gonist! – the more **A**s the better

**A**        **A**myloid vaccines – in the future!

# Substance dependence features

## Won't Resist Imbibing and Seeks Tipple Every Night

**W** **W**ithdrawal syndrome
**R** **R**einstatement (rapidly) of normal excessive intake after abstinence
**I** **I**nsight (subjective awareness) into compulsion for drug
**S** **S**alience (**P**rimacy or **P**rioritisation) of drinking over other activities
**T** **T**olerance development: ↑amounts needed
**E** **E**arly morning drink (is a type of 'relief')
**N** **N**arrowed repertoire: stereotyped drinking pattern

# Schneiderian first-rank symptoms

## Asking These Pleases Doctor Schneider

| | |
|---|---|
| **Asking** | **A**uditory hallucinations: 3 specific types as below[1] |
| **These** | **T**hought interference: 3 specific types as below[2] |
| **Pleases** | **P**assivity experiences: 3 specific types as below[3] |
| **Doctor** | **D**elusional perception[4] |
| **Schneider** | **S**omatic passivity[5] |

> 1 **Auditory hallucinations**: aren't first-rank symptoms unless they have ≥1 of 3 specific features which make the mnemonic '**EAR**':
> **E** **E**choes of own thoughts
> **A** **A**rguing (or discussing) voices of ≥2 people
> **R** **R**unning commentary on patient by the voices
> 2 **Thought interference**: insertion, broadcast or withdrawal of the patient's thoughts
> 3 **Passivity experiences** (= delusions of control): experiences that are 'made' or produced by an external force (ie not patient) and pertain to 3 specific types of experiences to make the mnemonic '**WEA**' (the record company):
> **W** **W**ill (= impulses)
> **E** **E**motions (= feelings or 'affect')
> **A** **A**ctions (volitional)
> 4 **Delusional perception**: attribution of unwarranted meaning to normal perception, eg 'The lights went green and suddenly I knew I was Jesus'
> 5 **Somatic passivity** (= delusion of alien penetration): feeling of part of the body or bodily function being controlled by an alien influence, ie not by the patient
>
> *This makes 11 first rank symptoms in total!*

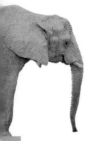

# 13. Haematology

rt 1

## Macrocytosis

rt 2

### My MIRACLE Diet Congenital Pregnancy

**My** **My**eloma, **My**elodysplastic/**My**eloproliferative disorders

**M** **M**yxoedema[1]
**I** **I**ntrinsic factor deficiency[2]
**R** **R**eticulocytosis[3]
**A** **A**ntivirals – especially **A**ZT (zidovudine)
**C** **C**ytotoxics[4]/COPD[5]
**L** **L**iver disease[6] (especially cirrhosis)
**E** **E**thanol[7] direct effects $\pm\downarrow B_{12}$/folate $\pm$liver disease

**Diet**[8]

**Congenital**[9]

**Pregnancy**: $\uparrow$ requirements of $B_{12}$/folate. Often mild

**notes**

1  Note that normocytic anaemia is more common in myxoedema
2  Pernicious anaemia most common cause. Others are gastrectomy, terminal ileal disease (eg Crohn's), atrophic gastritis and Zollinger–Ellison syndrome
3  Immature red cells released as a response to $\downarrow$ haematocrit
4  Not usually associated with anaemia. Causative agents include: azathioprine, methotrexate, hydroxyurea, cytosine, 6-mercaptopurine, cyclophosphamide. Other drugs (non-cytotoxics) include trimethoprim, OCP, biguanides, high-dose $K^+$ supplements
5  Caused by $CO_2$ retention leading to excess cell water retention
6  Caused by $\uparrow$cholesterol and phospholipids deposited in RBC membrane. Target cells also seen

notes

7 Direct effects of ethanol $\pm\downarrow B_{12}$/folate $\pm$liver disease
8 Dietary insufficiency of $B_{12}$ or folate. Can be malnutrition in the developing world but in developed countries is mostly vegans and alcoholics. Also remember rarer GI tract problems: malabsorption syndromes, small bowel overgrowth, (tropical) sprue, tapeworm, blind loop syndromes
9 Congenital causes, all rare: benign familial variants, Lesch–Nyhan syndrome, homocystinuria and folate enzyme deficiencies

## Secondary thrombocythaemia/ thrombocytosis

## HI PLATELETS

| | |
|---|---|
| **H** | **H**aemorrhage[1] |
| **I** | **I**nfection[2]/**I**nflammation[3] |
| **P** | **P**ost splenectomy (including ITP and hereditary spherocytosis) |
| **L** | **L**oss from urine: nephrotic/nephritic syndrome |
| **A** | **A**naemia[4] |
| **T** | **T**umour[5] |
| **E** | **E**thanol |
| **L** | **L**ow birth weight babies |
| **E** | **E**pinephrine/**E**xercise |
| **T** | **T**issue damage: trauma, surgery, burns or fractures |
| **S** | **S**ickle cell |

*HI covers the most common causes; **PLATELETS** covers the rarer causes*

notes

- **Secondary** (= **'Reactive'**) thrombocythemia is an exaggerated response to a primary condition, which is usually transient and resolves with this condition. Complications (thrombosis ± haemorrhage) are uncommon
- **Primary** (**'Essential'**) is autonomous production unregulated by physiological feedback. Causes are: PRV, familial essential polycythaemia, CML (rarely AML) and myelofibrosis with myeloid metaplasia. Complications (thrombosis ± haemorrhage) are more common

notes

1 If acute: ↑ release and ↑ production of platelets
2 Most severe infections: sepsis, meningitis, respiratory tract infections, UTIs, septic arthritis, osteomyelitis and gastroenteritis
3 Causes are '**I SHARK**':

   **I**   **I**nflammatory bowel disease

   **S**   **S**arcoid
   **H**   **H**enoch–Schönlein purpura
   **A**   **A**rthritis (rheumatoid)
   **R**   **R**heumatic fever
   **K**   **K** awasaki's
4 Fe deficiency (even if not due to bleeding) and less commonly haemolytic anaemias
5 Tumours: eg soft tissue sarcoma and osteosarcoma; chemotherapy can also cause this (eg vincristine)

## Eosinophilia

### AS PURE AS LIGHTS

**A**   **A**llergy: asthma/rhinitis/pneumonitis/drugs
**S**   **S**kin[1]: pemphig-**U**s (not –oid!)/**Ur**ticaria

**P**   **P**arasites[2]
**U**   **U**lcerative colitis
**R**   **R**adiation
**E**   **E**osinophilic granuloma[3]

**A**   **A**ddison's/**A**rteritis, eg polyarteritis nodosa, Churg–Strauss
**S**   **S**plenectomy

**L**   **L**oeffler's syndrome[4]/**L**oeffler's endocarditis[5]*
**I**   **I**nherited/**I**rradiation
**G**   **G**oodpasture's[6]
**H**   **H**ypereosinophilic syndrome[7]*
**T**   **T**umour: lymphoma (especially Hodgkin's), leukaemia (rarely)
**S**   **S**treptomycin[8]

*The first 3 in this list (AS P) are the most common causes!*

notes

1 Also occurs with common diseases such as eczema and psoriasis. Rarely Stevens–Johnson syndrome and dermatitis herpetiformis

2 Schistosomiasis, Echinococcosis and Helminths (Strongyloides, Ascariasis, Toxocariasis, Filariasis, Ankylostomiasis and Trichinosis)

3 1 of the 3 types** of histicytosis X: characterised by solitary bone lesions before adulthood. If pulmonary involvement (granulomas, cysts, bullae and eventually fibrosis ± spontaneous pneumothoraces), it is known as Langerhans cell histiocytosis

4 Aka 'pulmonary eosinophilia': cough + fever secondary to allergens; bugs (especially parasites such as *Ascaris lumbricoides*) + drugs. Transient reticular shadowing seen on CXR

5 Restrictive cardiomyopathy causing CCF and mitral regurgitation seen in temperate latitudes

6 Goodpasture's syndrome = autoantibodies against glomerular basement membrane causing vasculitis causing glomerulonephritis and pulmonary haemorrhage

7 >6 weeks of eosinophilia + systemic upset + end organ damage such as restrictive cardiomyopathy/pericarditis, neuropathy or hepatosplenomegaly. Often associated with myeloproliferative disorders or T cell lymphomas

8 Other drugs: penicillins

*Probably overlap as diseases
**Other 2 types are Letterer–Siwe disease (infant-onset fatal multisystem disease) and Hand–Schuller–Christian disease (young-onset diabetes insipidus, bony defects, exophthalmos and lung involvement)

---

**Part 1** Basophilia

---

**Part 2** ## MUMPS VIRUS

| | |
|---|---|
| **M** | **M**yeloproliferative diseases[1]/**M**alignancy in general |
| **U** | **U**C/**U**rticaria[2] |
| **M** | **M**yxoedema |
| **P** | **P**RV |
| **S** | **S**plenectomy |

**VIRUS**     Any viral infection – but particularly mumps!

notes

1 CML (if excessive may indicate transformation into accelerated or 'blastic' phase), PRV, myelofibrosis and essential thrombocythemia. Haemolysis is the other haematological cause

2 Including urticaria pigmentosa (= systemic mastocytosis)

# Basophilic stippling

## BASOPhilic

**B**   **B**eta (and other) thalassaemias
**A**   **A**naemia of chronic disease (is rare cause)
**S**   **S**ideroblastic anaemia
**O**   **O**ther dyserythropoietic anaemias
**P**   **P**b poisoning[1]

> **notes**
>
> Are dark granules (coarse punctate dots) in the RBC – condensed RNA in cytoplasm
>
> 1   This is known as an acquired sideroblastic anaemia. Less commonly caused by aluminium poisoning

# Dimorphic blood film

## TICS

**T**   **T**ransfusion[1]
**I**   **I**ron deficient anaemia[2]
**C**   **C**ombined iron and folate deficiency
**S**   **S**ideroblastic anaemia (primary)

> **notes**
>
> This is when 2 populations of blood cells exist simultaneously
>
> 1   Of patient with microcytosis or macrocytosis
> 2   That is being treated with iron

Hyposplenism

 **Medical[1] causes**

## GLASsES

| | |
|---|---|
| G | **G**liadin antibodies (= coeliac disease!) |
| L | **L**ymphoma/**L**eukaemia |
| A | **A**myloid |
| S | **S**ickle and thalassaemia |
| E | **E**arly life – neonates[2] |
| S | **S**LE |

**Features**

## SHAME

| | |
|---|---|
| S | **S**pherocytes[3] and Target cells (latter more common) |
| H | **H**owell–Jolly bodies[4] |
| A | **A**ntibiotic prophylaxis[5] needed if **A**splenia |
| M | **M** – Ig **M** levels decreased |
| E | **E**nhanced neutrophilia with infections |

---

1 Most common causes are surgical – following trauma or removal for haematological disease (ITP, malignancies and congenital haemolytic anaemias)
2 Congenital causes exist but are very rare
3 Often associated with anisocytosis (size) and poikilocytosis (shape) abnormalities
4 Nuclear remnants seen in RBC as blue dots – normally removed by spleen
5 Give life-long prophylactic penicillin V (phenoxymethylpenicillin) 250 mg bd. Also need vaccines for *S. pneumoniae* and *H. influenzae*

---

 Spherocytes

 **4Hs**

| | |
|---|---|
| H | **H**ereditary[1] |
| H | **H**aemolysis (autoimmune) |
| H | **H**yposplenism |
| H | **H**eat (= burns) |

---

1 Autosomal dominant transmission – linked to chromosome 8

# Target cells

## Iron SHOTS

**Iron** (ie Fe deficiency)

**S** **S**ickle
**H** **H**aemoglobin C[1] and D[2] disease
**O** **O**bstructive liver disease
**T** **T**halassaemias
**S** **S**plenectomy

*You put 'iron shot' in a gun when shooting at a target!*

> Cells look like targets, as the centre of the RBC is dark, surrounded by a pale middle section and then a dark rim
>
> 1 Genetic variant common in West Africa; homozygotes have more target cells than heterozygotes
> 2 Genetic variant causing haemolysis in homozygotes only

# Sideroblasts

## MARVEL LICE

**M** **M**yelodysplasia and **M**yeloproliferative disorders
**A** **A**ML
**R** **R**heumatoid arthritis (and connective tissue diseases)
**V** **V**asculitis
**E** **E**mbryonic: congenital (X-linked)
**L** **L**eukaemias (and carcinomatosis)

**L** **L**ead
**I** **I**soniazid
**C** **C**hloramphenicol
**E** **E**tOH

> Ring sideroblasts are precursors of red cells found in the bone marrow; they have peri-nuclear iron deposits seen as brown spots with Perl's iron stain

Leukoerythroblastic blood film

 **6Ms**

| | |
|---|---|
| M | **M**yelofibrosis |
| M | **M**yeloma |
| M | **M**yeloid leukaemia |
| M | **M**ets[1] in **M**arrow |
| M | **M**ycobacterium (TB) in **M**arrow |
| M | **M**assive haemorrhage |

> **notes**
>
> This is where immature red (normoblasts which still have their nucleus) and white (myelocytes and promyelocytes) cells are seen in the peripheral blood. Low Hb and platelets are often also seen, as well as a mild reticulocytosis
>
> 1 Especially from prostate, breast or lung cancer

**Part 1** Gaisbock's syndrome

**Part 2** **OBESE**

| | |
|---|---|
| O | **O**bese |
| B | **B**alding: middle aged |
| E | **E**levated Hb[1] and PCV[2] |
| S | **S**mokers |
| E | **E**pinephrine[3] |

> **notes**
>
> These patients are often overweight
>
> 1 Aka Gaisbock's polycythaemia
> 2 But normal red cell volume and ↓ plasma volume
> 3 Stressful occupations cause this: also aka 'Stress polycythaemia'

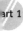

# Inherited thrombophilia (recurrent DVT)

## COLLAPSES

C **C**-protein deficiency[1]
O **O**estrogens[2]
L **L**upus anticoagulant (antiphospholipid syndrome)
L **L**eiden (factor V) mutation[3]
A **A**ntithrombin III[4]
P **P**rothrombin excess[5]/**P**NH[6]/**P**RV[7]
S **S**-protein deficiency[1]
E **E**rythrocytosis/**E**xcessive plasminogen activator inhibitor
S **S**ystinuria (ie homocystinuria!)

*Collapses occur due to PEs!*

> **notes**
>
> 1 Protein C deficiency is more common than protein S deficiency (hence its place higher up the list). Both are autosomal dominant deficiencies of vitamin-K-dependent factors that normally act together to inactivate factors V and VIII. *NB Risk of skin necrosis when protein-C-deficient patients started on anticoagulant therapy*
>
> 2 Any cause of elevated oestrogens will cause risk of thrombophilia, most of which are acquired (pregnancy, OCP, HRT) although some are inherited such as being female (!) and endocrine disorders
>
> 3 Factor V Leiden mutation is the commonest cause of activated protein C (APC) resistance and some estimates suggest 1 in 5 DVTs are caused by this mutation. Common (5% of healthy controls): screen all women for this if recurrent thrombosis (test for APC resistance) if starting combined OCP; risk seems to increase disproportionately with a combination of OCP and this disorder
>
> 4 Rare but causes very significant increase in risk of TE
>
> 5 Prothrombin excess: mutations to prothrombin gene are common and account for 20% of patients with venous thrombosis and a positive family history
>
> 6 Paroxysmal nocturnal haemoglobinuria
>
> 7 Polycythaemia rubra vera

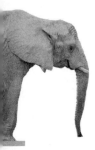

# 14. Therapeutics and toxicology

B$_1$ antagonists (selective)

## A BEAM

**A** **A**cebutolol
**B** **B**isoprolol (also Betaxolol but very rarely used)
**E** **E**smolol
**A** **A**tenolol
**M** **M**etoprolol

Cholinergic side-effects

## DUMBELS

**D** **D**iarrhoea
**U** **U**rination
**M** **M**iosis (constriction
**B** **B**ronchospasm/**B**radycardia
**E** **E**xcitation of CNS and muscle
**L** **L**acrimation
**S** **S**weating/**S**alivation

> In general they increase secretions*/fluid loss
>
> Commonly caused by Anticholinesterases which are either:
>
> - Peripherally acting: drugs for myasthenia, such as pyridostigmine or neostigmine. *This fact can be of use when trying to identify whether a patient with myasthenia is worsening due to a myasthenic crisis (will be dry) or over treatment with anticholinesterases
> - Centrally acting: drugs for Alzheimer's such as donepezil, rivastigmine and galantamine
>
> Anticholinergic (or more accurately anti-muscarinic) side-effects are of course the opposite of this and commonly caused by atropine/ipratropium, hyoscine as well as antihistamines, antipsychotics, antidepressants (especially tricyclics)

 **P450 inhibitors**

 **Heart and liver failure**

## OF DEVICES

| | |
|---|---|
| **O** | **O**meprazole |
| **F** | **F**luoxetine/**F**luvoxamine/**F**luconazole |
| | |
| **D** | **D**isulfiram |
| **E** | **E**rythromycin (and **C**larithromycin) |
| **V** | **V**alproate |
| **I** | **I**soniazid |
| **C** | **C**imetidine/**C**iprofloxacin |
| **E** | **E**tOH (acute abuse) |
| **S** | **S**ulphonamides |

> Commonly inhibited drugs: warfarin, phenytoin, carbamazepine, ciclosporin and theophyllines

# P450 inducers

## Cigarettes and alcohol

## PC BRAS

| | |
|---|---|
| **P** | **P**henytoin |
| **C** | **C**arbamazepine |
| | |
| **B** | **B**arbiturates (eg phenobarbital) |
| **R** | **R**ifampicin |
| **A** | **A**lcohol (chronic abuse) |
| **S** | **S**ulphonylureas/**St**. John's wort |

>  Commonly induced drugs: warfarin, phenytoin, carbamazepine, ciclosporin and theophyllines (as inhibitors) but also OCP

# Drug-induced SIADH

## 9Cs

| | |
|---|---|
| **C** | **C**ytotoxics[*1] (especially **C**yclophosphamide) |
| **C** | **C**hlorthalidone[*2] |
| **C** | **C**hlorpropamide |
| **C** | **C**hlormethiazole |
| **C** | **C**hlorpromazine[3] |
| **C** | **C**italopram[4] |
| **C** | **C**arbamazepine |
| **C** | **C**lofibrate |
| **C** | **C**igarettes (nicotine) |

>  *Most common causes
>
> Other causes include: lung or brain infections, trauma or tumour
>
> 1 Also vincristine and vinblastine
> 2 And other thiazides
> 3 And most other antipsychotics
> 4 And most other antidepressants: especially tricyclics

## Part 1 Fluoxetine side-effects

### FLUOXETINE

| | |
|---|---|
| **F** | **F**ever |
| **L** | **L**FT abnormalities |
| **U** | **U**lceration |
| **O** | **O**rgasm dysfunction (delay) |
| **X** | E**X**tra pyramidal side-effects |
| **E** | **E**cchymoses |
| **T** | **T**ension headaches* |
| **I** | **I**nsomnia* |
| **N** | **N**ausea* |
| **E** | **E**mesis/diarrhoea |

> *Most common

## Part 1 Antipsychotic side-effects

### TARDIVE

| | |
|---|---|
| **T** | **T**ardive dyskinesias*[1] |
| **A** | **A**granulocytosis[2] |
| **R** | **R**ash[3] |
| **D** | **D**ystonias (acute)*: eg oculogyric crisis |
| **I** | **I**nsulin resistance[4] |
| **V** | **V**entricular arrhythmias (secondary to ↑QT) |
| **E** | **E**ndocrine[5] |

> NB Also cause neuroleptic malignant syndrome which is easy to remember and therefore not included!
>
> 1 Mostly after chronic use but very rarely occurs after first dose: eg orofacial ("gurning")
> 2 Especially with clozapine
> 3 Any but also photosensitivity and contact dermatitis
> 4 Diabetes – especially with newer 'atypical' antipsychotics (which have serotonin, as well as dopamine, antagonism) such as olanzapine, risperidone, quetiapine and clozapine
> 5 Hyperprolactinaemia (due to dopamine antagonism): menstrual changes, infertility, galactorrhoea, sexual dysfunction and gynaecomastia (in men) and ↑weight
>
> *Are the most serious "Extrapyramidal side effects" – commonest is Parkinssonism

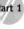

# Rifampicin

## 4Rs

| | |
|---|---|
| **R** | **R**evs up p450 (indexes) and LFTs (↑s) |
| **R** | **R**ed/orange secretions |
| **R** | **R**NA polymerase inhibitor |
| **R** | **R**apid **R**esistance if given on own |

# Drug-induced hepatitis

## FAT PINK CARS

| | |
|---|---|
| **F** | **F**e (iron salts) |
| **A** | **A**miodarone |
| **T** | **T**etracyclines |
| **P** | **P**yrazinamide |
| **I** | **I**soniazid |
| **N** | **N**itrofurantoin |
| **K** | **K**etoconazole (and other antifungals, especially Itraconazole) |
| **C** | **C**Cl$_4$ |
| **A** | **A**naesthetic agents (especially halothane) |
| **R** | **R**ifampicin |
| **S** | **S**tatins (HMG CoA inhibitors) |

*Paracetamol is considered too obvious to mention!*

NB Most drugs can cause hepatitis but the above are common causes and some of the most likely to cause severe hepatic impairment

# Lead poisoning

## ABCDEFGHIJK

| | |
|---|---|
| **A** | **A**naemia (mild but often symptomatic) |
| **B** | **B**asophilic stippling on blood film |
| **C** | **C**olic/**C**onstipation/**C**achexia |
| **D** | **D**ementia[1] |
| **E** | **E**ncephalitis/**E**ncephalopathy[1] |
| **F** | **F**oot (and wrist) drop: peripheral neuropathy[2] |

**G** **G**ingival hyperpigmentation[3]/**G**out-like symptoms/**G**onadal dysfunction

**H** **H**yperchloraemic acidosis (secondary to RTA)/**H**eadache/ **H**ypertension

**I** **I**nfertility/**I**nsomnia/**I**rritability

**J** **J**oint pains (arthralgia)

**K** **K**idney failure[4]

---

1 Occurs in severe cases
2 Motor involvement predominates; sensory involvement rare. Can also get optic nerve atrophy
3 Burton's lines: blue lines in gums
4 In acute poisoning causes ARF with ATN. If chronic causes Fanconi syndrome and interstitial nephritis

**Treatment**

- Remove source
- Chelating agents – penicillamine, succimer, edetate, dimercaprol

---

**Part 1** Myasthenia gravis exacerbators

**PACES** **Anti-cipate these drugs being dangerous before giving to someone with myasthenia!**

**Anti**biotics: especially **A**minoglycosides[1] and **Anti**malarials[2]
**Anti**depressants: **A**mitriptyline (and other tricyclics)
**Anti**psychotics: haloperidol and phenothiazines
**Anti**epileptics: phenytoin, carbamazepine, gabapentin
**Anti**hypertensives: beta-blockers* (including timolol eye drops)
**Anti**arrhythmics: verapamil*

---

**Penicillamine** (and interferon alpha) can *cause* the disease rather than *exacerbate* it! Intercurrent illness (and of course exercise – fatigability being the hallmark of the disease) can bring on symptoms. Neuromuscular blockers should be used cautiously

1 Gentamicin and other '-mycins'
2 Quinidine, quinine, chloroquine and tonic water

*These 2 cardiac drugs can be remembered as the 2 drugs not to be given together!

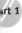

# Drug-induced lupus

## HIPPOPOTAMIS

| | |
|---|---|
| **H** | **H**ydralazine |
| **I** | **I**soniazid |
| **P** | **P**rocainamide |
| **P** | **P**enicillamine |
| **O** | **O**CP |
| **P** | **P**henylbutazone |
| **O** | **O**phthalmic timolol |
| **T** | **T**etracyclines (especially minocycline)/**T**NF/**T**iotropium |
| **A** | **A**nticonvulsants: valproate, carbamazepine, ethosuximide |
| **M** | **M**ethyldopa |
| **I** | **I**nterleukins/**I**nterferons |
| **S** | **S**ulphonamides/**S**tatins (simva/lova)/**S**ulfasalazine |

*Hippo (especially Hip) covers the most common causes*

> **notes**
>
> NB Often resolve if drug(s) stopped
>
> Penicillins, hydrochlorothiazide can cause flares of SLE but not cause it!
>
> Differences to *non-drug induced* lupus:
>
> - Anti-histone antibodies are very common (95%)
> - Low incidence of anti-Sm and anti-ds DNA positivity
> - Normal sex ratio (not increased in females)
> - Little CNS or renal involvement
> - Increased risk if low acetylators (or HLA-DR3 positive)

# Lithium toxicity

## Core features

| | |
|---|---|
| **C** | **C**erebellar signs (**C**oordination loss, etc) |
| **C** | **C**oarse tremor (NB fine tremor is side-effect!) |
| **C** | **C**onfusion |
| **C** | **C**onvulsion |
| **C** | **C**irculatory failure (renal failure secondary to this or other cause?) |
| **C** | **C**ollapse |
| **C** | **C**oma |
| **C** | **C**orpse |

### Danger of renal failure/toxicity if . . .

**D** **D**iuretics (especially thiazides)
**D** **D**ehydration (including diarrhoea and vomiting)
**D** **D**ietary **D**eficiency of Na (↑ renal Na therefore Li retention)

## Serotonin syndrome

### SEROTONIN

**S** **S**weating
**E** **E**pileptic fits
**R** **R**andom speech (confusion)
**O** **O**verheating
**T** **T**remor
**O** **O**ccasional spasms (myoclonus)
**N** **N**ystagmus
**I** **I**rritability
**N** **N**asty rhythms (arrhythmias)

> **notes**
>
> Serotonin syndrome can occur with any drug that upregulates 5-HT leading to dangerously high levels. MAOIs are particularly notorious for this, especially if used with other potent upregulators such as SSRIs (which are contraindicated with them) or if tryptophan-rich foods are ingested at the same time. Also occurs with interactions which increase antidepressant levels

## SSRI discontinuation (withdrawal) syndrome

### Suddenly Stopping Five-HT Drugs Precipitates Agitation

| | |
|---|---|
| **Suddenly** | **S**quits (= diarrhoea!) |
| **Stopping** | **S**hock-like sensations ('electric') |
| **Five HT** | **F**lu-like symptoms |
| **Drugs** | **D**izziness |
| **Precipitates** | **P**araesthesia |
| **Agitation** | **A**gitation |

> **notes**
>
> SSRI discontinuation syndrome occurs on stopping SSRIs suddenly – this is why it is essential to tell patients on SSRIs not to stop the medications themselves and if they wish to stop to consult a doctor. The likelihood of this occurring is related to (amongst other things) the half-life of the SSRI in question – the shorter the half-life, the more likely it is to occur – therefore it is most likely to occur with paroxetine (and least likely with fluoxetine)

## Benzodiazepine withdrawal syndrome

### Suddenly Stopping Benzos Makes People Have Rebound Anxiety

| | |
|---|---|
| **Suddenly** | **S**leeplessness |
| **Stopping** | **S**hakiness |
| **Benzos** | **B**uzzing in ear (tinnitus) |
| **Makes** | **M**etal taste |
| **People** | **P**erceptual changes |
| **Have** | **H**eadache |
| **Rebound** | **R**estlessness |
| **Anxiety** | **A**nxiety |

> **notes**
>
> Benzodiazepine withdrawal occurs on stopping benzodiazepines too quickly. This is more likely (and more severe) if the half-life of the benzodiazepine is short; therefore, when stopping benzodiazepines convert to a long-acting drug such as diazepam. To minimise the risk of withdrawal symptoms reduce the dose by one-eighth every 2 weeks

Part 1

# Lithium side-effects

Part 2

## D and Ts

### Early effects

**D**   **D**iarrhoea: also nausea and vomiting
**T**   **T**hirst
**T**   **T**iredness/fatigue (including muscular weakness)
**T**   **T**aste disturbance (metallic)
**T**   **T**remor (fine – note coarse tremor occurs in toxicity)

### Late effects

**D**   **D**iabetes insipidus
**T**   **T**hyroid dysfunction (mostly decrease but can increase)
**T**   **T** wave flattening and arrhythmias
**T**   **T**ardive dyskinesia
**T**   **T**eenage skin (acne!)

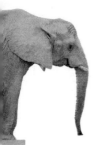

# 15. Infectious diseases

Part 1

## Strongyloides

Part 2

### Strong ALES

#### Strong

| | |
|---|---|
| A | **A**sthma-like presentation[1] |
| L | **L**arva currens[2] |
| E | **E**osinophilia/**E**nteral malabsorption |
| S | **S**ystemic (and **S**tomach) upset[3] |

*Think of someone who spends too much time drinking strong ales; abdominal pains and itching from liver damage and wheezy from smoking!*

>
>
> Infections are caused by the filariform nematode *Strongyloides stercoralis*: most infections are *asymptomatic*, unless immunocompromised when 'hyperinfection syndrome' is more likely (multisystem illness suggestive of pneumonia, meningitis ±sepsis)
>
> #### Diagnosis
>
> - Eosinophilia, serology, stool microscopy and culture (sputum or duodenal aspirate samples can also contain larvae). CXR can show pulmonary infiltrates
>
> #### Treatment
>
> - Thiabendazole or albendazole (fewer side-effects); avoid steroids for 'asthma' (can worsen)

**notes**

1 Wheeze and cough due to 'eosinophilic pneumonitis'
2 Larva currens* = cutaneous migration of larvae ⇒ pruritic "serpiginous" rash with raised wheal and surrounding flare (ie urticarial); common on trunk and buttocks. Migration is quick (cm/h); comes and goes quickly (ie over hours). On initial infection erythematous itchy papules occur as the skin is penetrated by larvae
3 Fever is common, as are pains, diarrhoea, vomiting and fever

*NB Not to be confused with larva **migrans**, which occurs with *Ancylostoma braziliense* (hookworm found in cats and dogs) that causes peripheral rash with no surrounding erythema. More stable over time (lasts weeks) and migrates more slowly (cm/day). Larvae cannot leave subcutaneous tissues in humans and bury around skin; red papules just behind larva followed by red raised track (especially feet). Treatment: thiabendazole (topical) and albendazole (by mouth)

**Part 1**

# AIDS-defining illnesses

**Part 2**

HIV-positive plus one or more of:

## CRIPTOCOCCS

| | |
|---|---|
| **C** | *Cryptococcus neoformans* infections |
| **R** | **R**etinal toxoplasmosis[1] (**C**erebral abscess more common though) |
| **I** | **I**nvasive cervical carcinoma |
| **P** | **P**CP (*Pneumocystis carinii* pneumonia) |
| **T** | **T**B: pulmonary, extrapulmonary or disseminated (*M. avium*) |
| **O** | **O**esophageal, pulmonary or disseminated (*not oral*) *Candida*[2] |
| **C** | *Cryptosporidium*[3] ⇒ diarrhoea for >1 month |
| **O** | **O**ral leukoplakia |
| **C** | **C**MV activation: retinitis, cholangitis, colitis/oesophagitis[4] and encephalitis |
| **C** | **C**occidioidomycosis (extrapulmonary) |
| **S** | **S**almonella septicaemia – recurrent |

NB This list is not exhaustive!

notes

1 Toxoplasmosis can also rarely cause myocarditis and pneumonitis

NB CMV retinitis is a differential diagnosis of retinitis in HIV (first narrowing of vessels, then vascular occlusion and perivascular haemorrhages causing red 'ketchup' areas and retinal ischaemia (white areas)). Treatment: iv ganciclovir

2 Not oral: gastric washing shows hyphae. Treatment: fluconazole/nystatin
3 *Cryptosporidium*. Diagnosis: look for red cysts on Ziehl–Nielsen stain. Treatment (for resistance cases): spiramycin and paromomycin
4 CMV in GI $\Rightarrow$ round intranuclear inclusion bodies in epithelial cells of mucosa

---

# False-positive VDRL

## SYPHILITIC

**S**   **S**LE (including antiphospholipid syndrome)/**S**jögren's
**Y**   **Y**aws*
**P**   **P**inta*
**H**   **H**ashimoto's/**H**epatitis A/**H**aemolytic anaemias
**I**   **I**nfective endocarditis
**L**   **L**eprosy/**L**eptospirosis
**I**   **I**nfective malaria
**T**   **T**B
**I**   **I**nfectious mononucleosis (EBV)
**C**   **C**ronies (old age!)

notes

*Other Treponemal spp diseases

VDRL is not a specific test but good marker of activity; reduces in 'latent period' between the secondary (rash stage) and tertiary (gumma stage) stages

Note TPHA (Treponema Pallidum Haem Agglutinin) test is more specific

FTA (fluorescent treponemal antibody) most useful in congenital cases and is the most specific

Secondary syphilis:

- Rash (hand, feet ±trunk, legs, face)
- Meningitis
- Oropharynx
- Other: kidney, GI/liver, bones/joints

Part 1 Whipple's disease

Part 2 **WHIP LASH**

W **W**eight loss (malabsorption syndrome)
H **H**yperpigmentation
I **I**ntestinal upset[1]
P **P**leurisy* (and cough)

L **L**ymphadenopathy (±hepatosplenomegaly)
A **A**rthritis*[2]/**A**naemia
S **S**ystemic upset*: malaise/fever/cough
H **H**eart dysfunction: valve lesions (especially left-sided) and pericarditis**
E **E**ye signs (ophthalmoplegia/scotoma/uveitis)
S **S**eizures[3]

---

Whipple's disease is a rare disease caused by *Tropheryma whippelli* infection

1 Abdominal pains and diarrhoea (including steatorrhoea) common
2 Migratory polyarthritis (especially ankle/knee initially) or sacroiliitis
3 Almost any other neurological symptom/sign can occur: most common/important are meningitis, facial myoclonus, hypothalamic syndrome (insomnia, hyperphagia, polydipsia)

*Early symptoms; often non-specific leading to diagnostic delay. Other features can take many years to develop!
**Can reflect more generalised serositis

### Diagnosis

● Jenunal biopsy; intact villi but cells of lamina propria are replaced by macrophages containing PAS +ve glycoprotein granules – similar cells seen in spleen, lymph nodes and liver. PCR of biopsy is definitive test.

### Treatment

● Penicillin (im) and streptomycin followed after 2 weeks by co-trimoxazole (po) for 1 year – relapse common

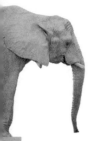

# 16. Genetics

rt 1

## X-linked recessive disorders

rt 2

### Fortunately Males Have Less Number of X Chromosome

| | |
|---|---|
| **Fortunately** | **F**ragile X syndrome |
| **Males** | **M**uscular dystrophies (Becker's/Duchenne's)/ **M**enke's |
| **Have** | **H**unter's syndrome |
| **Less** | **L**esch–Nyhan |
| **Number** | **N**ephrogenic diabetes insipidus |
| **Of** | **O**culocerebrorenal syndrome |
| **X** | **X**mas (Christmas!) disease = haemophilias |
| **Chromosome** | **C**erebellar ataxia (SCAs) |

rt 1

## Autosomal dominant disorders

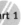

rt 2

### CAVE MAN TRAPS

| | |
|---|---|
| C | **C**rouzon syndrome |
| A | **A**pert's syndrome |
| V | **V**on–Hippel–Lindau (VHL) disease |
| E | **E**ndocrine disorders (MEN) |
| M | **M**yotonic dystrophy |
| A | **A**crocephalosyndactyly |
| N | **N**eurofibromatosis (types I and II |
| T | **T**reacher Collins / Tay-Sachs |
| R | **R**otor |
| A | **A**cute intermittent porphyria |
| P | **P**hacomatoses: tuberous sclerosis, neurofibromatosis, VHL, Sturge–Weber |
| S | **S**turge–Weber |

# X-linked dominant disorders

## CV RIP

**C**   **C**hronic granulomatous disease
**V**   **V**itamin-D-resistant rickets

**R**   **R**ett's syndrome
**I**   **I**ncontinentia pigmentii
**P**   **P**seudo-hypoparathyroidism

All other common genetic conditions, by exclusion, are autosomal recessive!

# Mnemonic index

TINS OF PEACH  82–3
TROPICAL ZOO  30

ULCER  53

VOMED  45

WE RANK MAN  56–7
WHIP LASHES  128
Won't Resist Imbibing and
      Seeks Tipple Every Night
      103
WRITHES ABOUT A LOT  70–1

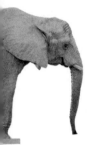

# Subject index